SIMPLE & Delicious

Healthy Recipes from the Better Care Kitchen

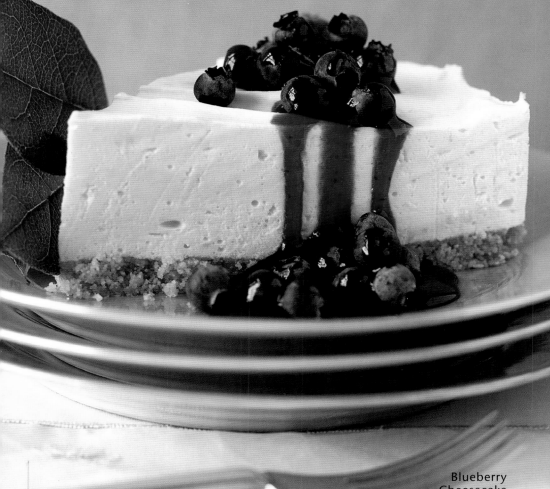

Blueberry
Cheesecake
page 107

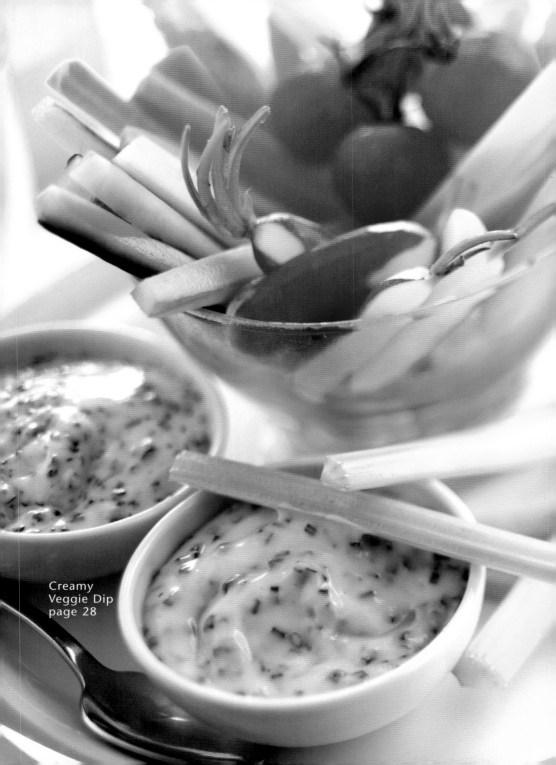

Creamy
Veggie Dip
page 28

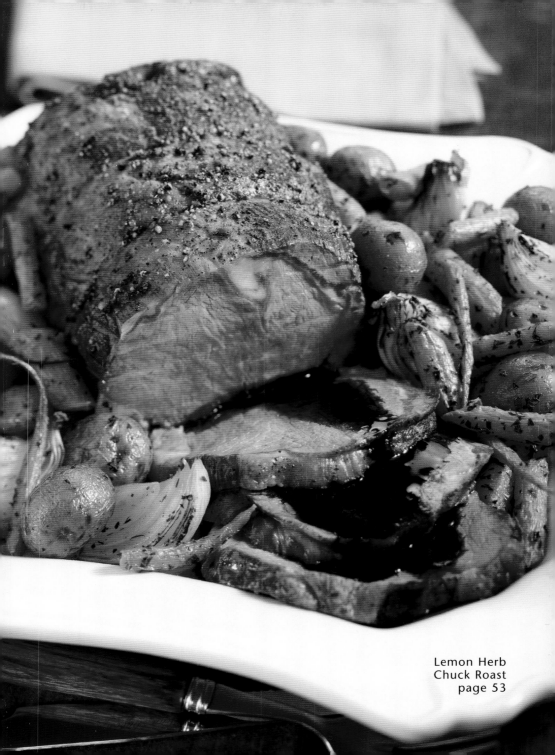

Lemon Herb
Chuck Roast
page 53

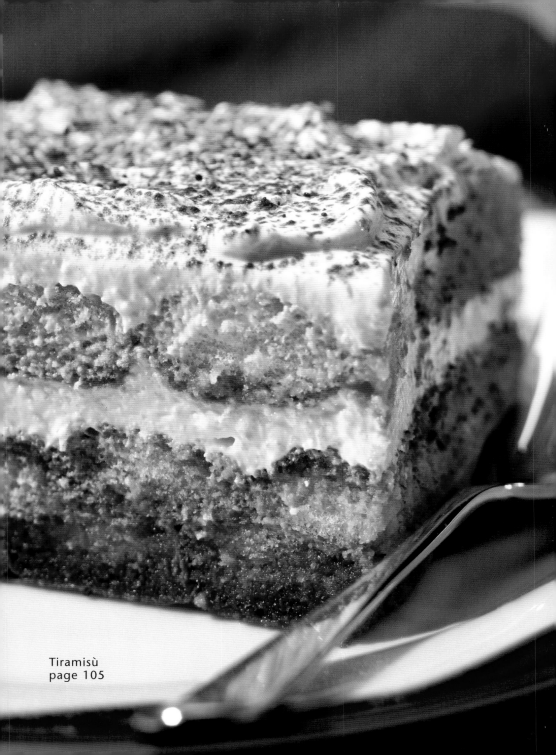

Tiramisù
page 105

SIMPLE & Delicious

Healthy Recipes from the Better Care Kitchen

Published by AmMed Direct
Copyright ©2007

AmMed Direct
P.O. Box 290309
Nashville, Tennessee 37229-0309
800.435.1458
www.AmMedDirect.com

AmMed HomeCare Pharmacy
800.282.3524

Food Photography: pages 2, 3, 4, 15, 16, 49, 85 © by Food Image Source; cover and pages 13, 14, 50, 51, 52, 86, 87, 88 © by FoodPix

Dietary Exchanges and Carbohydrate Choices: AmMed Direct

ISBN-10: 0-9778333-0-5
ISBN-13: 978-0-9778333-0-6

Edited, Designed, and Manufactured by
Favorite Recipes® Press
An imprint of

FRP

P.O. Box 305142
Nashville, Tennessee 37230
800.358.0560

Art Director: Steve Newman
Book Design: Starletta Polster
Project Manager and Editor: Debbie Van Mol, RD

Printed in China
First Printing 2007   30,000 copies
Second Printing 2007   15,000 copies
Third Printing 2008   25,000 copies
Fourth Printing 2008   10,000 copies

Table of Contents

Desserts 84

Dedication

This cookbook is dedicated

to the valued members

in the Better Care Program™.

We are so glad

to have you with us!

Dear Friend,

You are holding in your hands a gift to you from our Better Care Program™. This program, and this cookbook, were created specifically to help make your life with diabetes easier.

We understand diabetes requires important medical testing and education to help you avoid or reduce other health complications. As part of our commitment to you, we designed this cookbook to help you do just that.

Most individuals with diabetes often ask, "What can I eat?" Our editors have hand-selected the recipes in this book just for you. They have all been reviewed by a registered dietitian to ensure they meet healthful eating guidelines for persons with diabetes.

Below each recipe you'll find the nutritional information per serving to help you stay within the daily meal plan that works for you. Best of all, our editors have also made sure these recipes are relatively simple, flavorful, and enjoyable to eat!

We're so glad you are a member of AmMed Direct's Better Care Program™! We gratefully dedicate this cookbook to you.

Sincerely,

Tom Milam
General Manager
AmMed Direct

Nutritional Profile Guidelines

The editors have attempted to present these family recipes in a format that allows approximate nutritional values to be computed. Persons with dietary or health problems or whose diets require close monitoring should not rely solely on the nutritional information provided. They should consult their physician or a registered dietitian for specific information.

ABBREVIATIONS FOR NUTRITIONAL PROFILE

carb—carbohydrate   g—grams   mg—milligrams

Nutritional information for these recipes is computed from information derived from many sources, including materials supplied by the United States Department of Agriculture, computer databanks, and journals in which the information is assumed to be in the public domain. However, many specialty items, new products, and processed foods may not be available from these sources or may vary from the average values used in these profiles. More information on new and/or specific products may be obtained by reading the nutrient labels. Unless otherwise specified, the nutritional profile of these recipes is based on all measurements being level.

- Artificial sweeteners vary in use and strength and should be used to taste, using the recipe ingredients as a guideline. Sweeteners using aspartame (NutraSweet and Equal) should not be used as sweeteners in recipes involving prolonged heating, which reduces the sweet taste. For further information on the use of these sweeteners, refer to the package.

- Alcoholic ingredients have been analyzed for the basic information. Cooking causes the evaporation of alcohol, which decreases alcoholic and caloric content.
- Buttermilk, sour cream, and yogurt are the types available commercially.
- Canned beans and vegetables have been analyzed along with their canning liquid. Draining and rinsing canned products will reduce the sodium content.
- Chicken, cooked for boning and chopping, has been roasted; this cooking method yields the lowest caloric values.
- Eggs are all large. If you are concerned about using raw eggs that may carry salmonella, as in eggnog, use eggs pasteurized in their shells, which are sold at some specialty food stores, or use an equivalent amount of pasteurized egg substitute.
- Flour is unsifted all-purpose flour.
- Garnishes, serving suggestions, and other optional information and variations are not included in the profile.
- Margarine and butter are regular, not whipped or presoftened.
- Oil is any type of vegetable cooking oil. Shortening is hydrogenated vegetable shortening.
- Salt and other ingredients to taste as noted in the ingredients have not been included in the nutritional profile.
- If a choice of ingredients has been given, the profile reflects the first option. If a choice of amounts has been given, the profile reflects the greater amount.
- The nutritional analysis for each recipe represents one serving size. Eating two servings doubles all of the nutritional values.

Snacks Contents

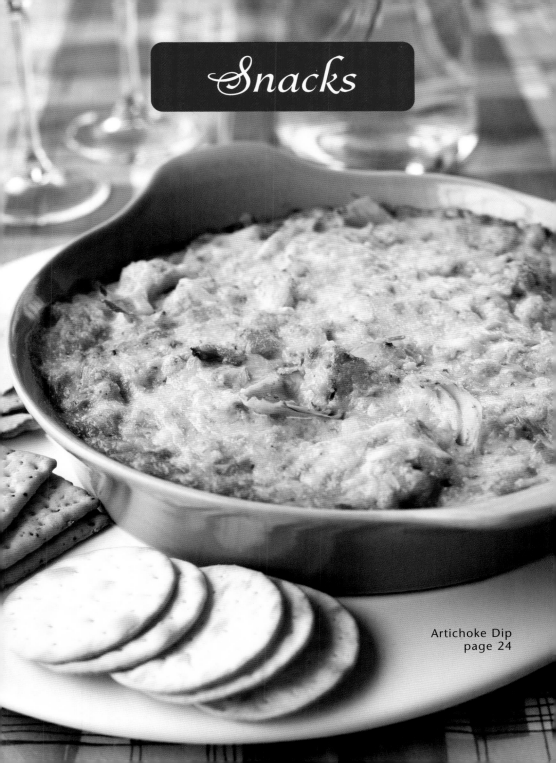

Snacks

Artichoke Dip
page 24

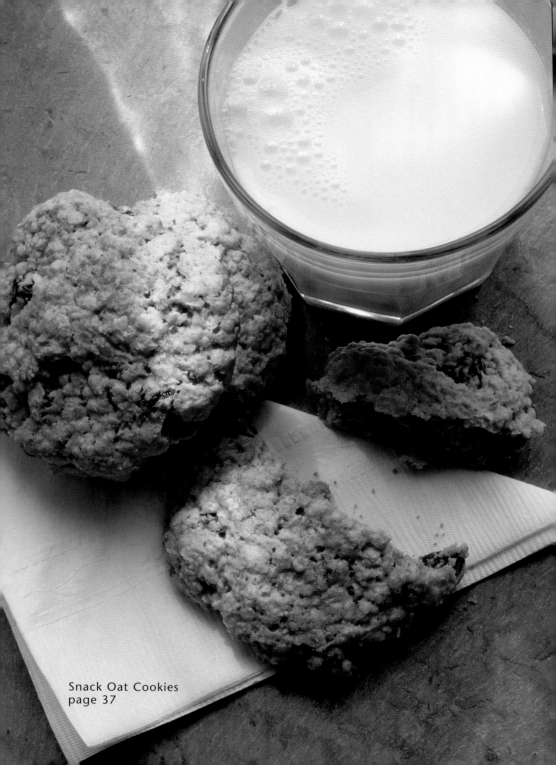

Snack Oat Cookies
page 37

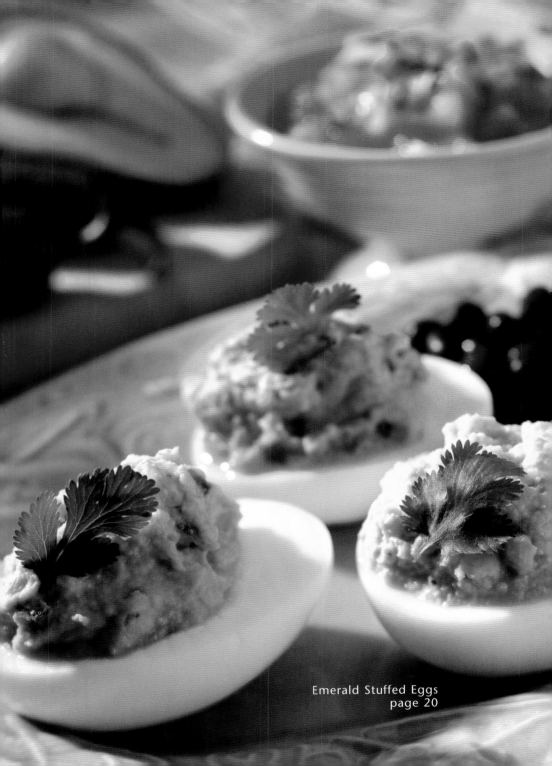

Emerald Stuffed Eggs
page 20

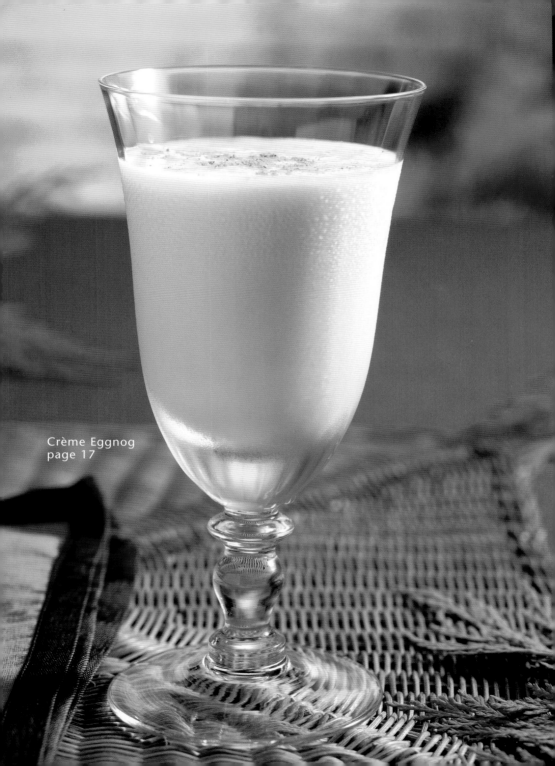

Crème Eggnog
page 17

Crème Eggnog

PHOTOGRAPH FOR THIS RECIPE APPEARS ON PAGE 16.

1 (7-ounce) jar marshmallow creme
1 cup skim milk
2 cups liquid egg substitute
1 teaspoon vanilla extract
Rum extract to taste
8 ounces nonfat whipped topping
Ground nutmeg to taste

Spoon the marshmallow creme into a mixing bowl and add the skim milk gradually, beating constantly until smooth. Beat in the egg substitute until blended and stir in the flavorings. Fold in the whipped topping. Chill, covered, until serving time. Spoon into stemmed goblets and sprinkle with nutmeg. Serve immediately.

Yield: 10 servings

NUTRIENTS PER SERVING

Calories	154	Cholesterol	1 mg	Fiber	0 g
Total Fat	2 g	Protein	7 g	Sodium	128 mg
Saturated Fat	<1 g	Carbohydrates	26 g	Total Sugar	17 g

DIETARY EXCHANGES: 2 Other Carbohydrate/Sugar
CARB CHOICES: 2

WHAT LIES BEHIND US AND WHAT LIES BEFORE US ARE TINY MATTERS COMPARED TO WHAT LIES WITHIN US.

—RALPH WALDO EMERSON

Frosty Nog

1 pint frozen vanilla yogurt
2 cups skim milk
$1^1/2$ to 2 tablespoons rum extract
Ground nutmeg to taste

Combine the yogurt, skim milk, flavoring and nutmeg in a blender and process until smooth. Pour into chilled mugs and serve immediately.

Yield: 8 servings

NUTRIENTS PER SERVING

Calories	100	Cholesterol	3 mg	Fiber	0 g
Total Fat	<1 g	Protein	5 g	Sodium	49 mg
Saturated Fat	<1 g	Carbohydrates	18 g	Total Sugar	12 g

DIETARY EXCHANGES: 1 Milk
CARB CHOICES: 1

HAPPINESS IS NOT A DESTINATION. IT IS A METHOD OF LIFE.

—BURTON HILLS

Rosemary-Toasted Pecans

1 egg white
3 cups pecan halves
4 teaspoons minced fresh rosemary, or
  2 teaspoons dried rosemary
$1/2$ teaspoon salt
$1/2$ teaspoon freshly ground pepper

Preheat the oven to 350 degrees. Line the bottom of a 9×13-inch baking dish with foil and spray lightly with nonstick cooking spray. Beat the egg white in a mixing bowl until frothy.

Add the pecans to the egg white and toss to coat. Stir in a mixture of the rosemary, salt and pepper. Spread the pecans in a single layer in the prepared baking dish and toast for 15 to 20 minutes or until light brown. Remove to a platter to cool.

Yield: 12 (1/4-cup) servings

NUTRIENTS PER SERVING

Calories	189	Cholesterol	0 mg	Fiber	3 g
Total Fat	19 g	Protein	3 g	Sodium	102 mg
Saturated Fat	2 g	Carbohydrates	4 g	Total Sugar	1 g

DIETARY EXCHANGES: 4 Fat
CARB CHOICES: 0

Emerald Stuffed Eggs

PHOTOGRAPH FOR THIS RECIPE APPEARS ON PAGE 15.

1 (10-ounce) package frozen chopped spinach
12 hard-cooked eggs, peeled
$1/2$ cup light mayonnaise
2 tablespoons grated Parmesan cheese
Salt and freshly ground pepper to taste
Flat-leaf parsley for garnish

Cook the spinach using the package directions. Drain and press the excess moisture from the spinach. Cut the eggs lengthwise into halves and remove the yolks to a bowl, reserving the whites. Mash the egg yolks.

Add the spinach, mayonnaise, cheese, salt and pepper to the egg yolks and mix well. Mound the spinach mixture in the reserved egg whites and arrange on a platter. Garnish each stuffed egg with flat-leaf parsley. Chill, covered, until serving time.

Yield: 24 ($1/2$-egg) servings

NUTRIENTS PER SERVING

Calories	61	Cholesterol	108 mg	Fiber	<1 g
Total Fat	5 g	Protein	4 g	Sodium	86 mg
Saturated Fat	1 g	Carbohydrates	1 g	Total Sugar	1 g

DIETARY EXCHANGES: 1 Lean Meat
CARB CHOICES: 0

Cheese-Stuffed Tomatoes

15 cherry tomatoes
$1/2$ cup 2% cottage cheese
1 tablespoon thinly sliced green onion
$1/2$ teaspoon minced fresh dill weed, or
   $1/8$ teaspoon dried dill weed
$1/8$ teaspoon lemon pepper

Cut a thin slice off the bottom of each tomato. Scoop out the pulp with a small melon baller, discarding the pulp. Invert the tomatoes on a wire rack to drain.

Combine the cottage cheese, green onion, dill weed and lemon pepper in a bowl and mix well. Spoon the cottage cheese mixture into the tomatoes. Serve immediately or store, covered, in the refrigerator for up to 8 hours.

Yield: 15 tomatoes

NUTRIENTS PER TOMATO

Calories	11	Cholesterol	1 mg	Fiber	<1 g
Total Fat	<1 g	Protein	1 g	Sodium	36 mg
Saturated Fat	<1 g	Carbohydrates	1 g	Total Sugar	<1 g

DIETARY EXCHANGES: Free
CARB CHOICES: 0

THERE ARE TWO WAYS OF MEETING DIFFICULTIES: YOU ALTER THE DIFFICULTIES, OR YOU ALTER YOURSELF TO MEET THEM.

—PHYLLIS BOTTOME

Zucchini and Blue Cheese Roll-Ups

3 ounces light cream cheese, softened
2 ounces blue cheese, crumbled
$1/2$ cup finely chopped walnuts
4 (6-ounce) zucchini

Mix the cream cheese and blue cheese in a bowl with a fork until blended. Stir in $1/3$ cup of the walnuts. Cut the zucchini into thirty-two paper-thin 1-inch-wide strips using a vegetable peeler or sharp knife.

Spoon approximately $1/2$ teaspoon of the cheese mixture onto one end of each strip and roll to enclose the filling. Dip one end of each roll-up in the remaining walnuts. Arrange walnut side up on a serving plate. Chill, covered, for 1 hour or until firm.

Yield: 32 roll-ups

NUTRIENTS PER ROLL-UP

Calories	26	Cholesterol	2 mg	Fiber	<1 g
Total Fat	2 g	Protein	1 g	Sodium	37 mg
Saturated Fat	1 g	Carbohydrates	1 g	Total Sugar	1 g

DIETARY EXCHANGES: Free
CARB CHOICES: 0

Citrus Cranberry Relish

2 oranges
2 Granny Smith apples, cored
1 (12-ounce) package fresh cranberries
18 envelopes Splenda

Peel the oranges, reserving the peel from one orange. Process the reserved peel in a food processor until finely chopped. Seed the oranges and process the oranges, apples and cranberries separately in a food processor until coarsely chopped.

Combine the chopped orange peel, chopped oranges, chopped apples, chopped cranberries and artificial sweetener in a bowl and mix well. Chill, covered, for 24 hours before serving.

Yield: 11 (^{1}/2-cup) servings

NUTRIENTS PER SERVING

Calories	43	Cholesterol	0 mg	Fiber	3 g
Total Fat	<1 g	Protein	<1 g	Sodium	1 mg
Saturated Fat	<1 g	Carbohydrates	11 g	Total Sugar	7 g

DIETARY EXCHANGES: 1 Fruit
CARB CHOICES: 1

LAUGHTER IS THE CLOSEST DISTANCE BETWEEN TWO PEOPLE.

Artichoke Dip

PHOTOGRAPH FOR THIS RECIPE APPEARS ON PAGE 13.

1 cup nonfat cottage cheese
2 tablespoons chopped fresh chives
2 tablespoons skim milk
$1/4$ teaspoon basil
$1/4$ teaspoon seasoned salt
Tabasco sauce to taste
Garlic powder to taste
3 or 4 canned artichoke hearts, drained,
   rinsed and finely chopped
2 tablespoons grated Parmesan cheese

Combine the cottage cheese, chives, skim milk, basil, seasoned salt, Tabasco sauce and garlic powder in a blender or food processor and process until smooth. Mix the cottage cheese mixture, artichokes and Parmesan cheese in a bowl and chill, covered, for 4 hours or longer. Serve with assorted party crackers or fresh vegetables.

Yield: 14 servings

NUTRIENTS PER SERVING

Calories	25	Cholesterol	1 mg	Fiber	<1 g
Total Fat	<1 g	Protein	3 g	Sodium	173 mg
Saturated Fat	<1 g	Carbohydrates	3 g	Total Sugar	1 g

DIETARY EXCHANGES: Free
CARB CHOICES: 0

Texas Caviar

1 (15-ounce) can hominy, drained and rinsed
1 (14-ounce) can black-eyed peas,
    drained and rinsed
1 cup picante sauce
2 tomatoes, chopped and drained
1 green bell pepper, chopped
1 small white onion, finely chopped
2 green onions, sliced
2 garlic cloves, minced
$1/4$ cup chopped fresh cilantro or parsley
Paprika to taste

Combine the hominy, black-eyed peas, picante sauce, tomatoes, bell pepper, white onion, green onions and garlic in a bowl and mix well. Chill, covered, in the refrigerator. Stir in the cilantro and sprinkle with paprika just before serving. Serve with baked tortilla chips.

Yield: 14 ($1/2$-cup) servings

NUTRIENTS PER SERVING

Calories	60	Cholesterol	<1 mg	Fiber	3 g
Total Fat	1 g	Protein	2 g	Sodium	242 mg
Saturated Fat	<1 g	Carbohydrates	12 g	Total Sugar	2 g

DIETARY EXCHANGES: 2 Vegetable
CARB CHOICES: 1

A FRIEND IS SOMEONE WITH WHOM YOU DARE TO BE YOURSELF.

—FRANK CRANE

Beefy Salsa Dip

8 ounces ground round
1 envelope taco seasoning mix
8 ounces low-fat cream cheese, softened
1 (15-ounce) can fat-free refried beans
2 cups fresh salsa
8 ounces low-fat Cheddar cheese, shredded
2 green onions, chopped

Preheat the oven to 350 degrees. Brown the beef in a skillet, stirring until crumbly; drain. Stir in the seasoning mix.

Layer the cream cheese, refried beans, beef mixture and salsa in a 9-inch baking dish. Sprinkle with the cheese and bake for 20 minutes or until the cheese melts. Sprinkle with the green onions and serve with baked tortilla chips.

Yield: 24 (^{1}/4-cup) servings

NUTRIENTS PER SERVING

Calories	81	Cholesterol	13 mg	Fiber	1 g
Total Fat	4 g	Protein	6 g	Sodium	225 mg
Saturated Fat	2 g	Carbohydrates	5 g	Total Sugar	<1 g

DIETARY EXCHANGES: 1 Medium Fat Meat, 1 Vegetable
CARB CHOICES: 0

Italian Tuna Dip

1 (6-ounce) can water-pack white tuna, drained
1 envelope Italian salad dressing mix
1 cup light sour cream

Flake the tuna in a bowl and stir in the salad dressing mix and sour cream. Chill, covered, for 8 hours. Serve with baked chips or melba rounds.

Yield: 12 servings

NUTRIENTS PER SERVING

Calories	51	Cholesterol	13 mg	Fiber	0 g
Total Fat	2 g	Protein	5 g	Sodium	247 mg
Saturated Fat	1 g	Carbohydrates	3 g	Total Sugar	3 g

DIETARY EXCHANGES: 1 Medium Fat Protein
CARB CHOICES: 0

IF YOU LOVE SOMEBODY, LET THEM GO,
FOR IF THEY RETURN, THEY ARE ALWAYS YOURS.
AND IF THEY DON'T, THEY NEVER WERE.

—KAHLIL GIBRAN

Creamy Veggie Dip

PHOTOGRAPH FOR THIS RECIPE APPEARS ON PAGE 2.

$1/2$ cup reduced-fat mayonnaise
$1/2$ cup 2% cottage cheese
$1/2$ cup plain low-fat yogurt
1 to 2 tablespoons minced onion
1 teaspoon parsley flakes
2 teaspoons dill weed
Salt to taste

Combine the mayonnaise, cottage cheese, yogurt, onion, parsley flakes, dill weed and salt in a bowl and mix well. Chill, covered, until serving time. Serve with cherry tomatoes, celery sticks, carrot sticks and/or radishes.

Yield: 12 servings

NUTRIENTS PER SERVING

Calories	32	Cholesterol	1 mg	Fiber	<1 g
Total Fat	2 g	Protein	2 g	Sodium	132 mg
Saturated Fat	1 g	Carbohydrates	3 g	Total Sugar	1 g

DIETARY EXCHANGES: 1 Very Lean Protein
CARB CHOICES: 0

Peanut Caramel Dunk

$1/4$ cup reduced-fat peanut butter
2 tablespoons fat-free caramel topping
2 tablespoons skim milk
2 apples, thinly sliced

Combine the peanut butter, caramel topping and skim milk in a small saucepan. Cook over low heat until heated through, stirring constantly. Serve warm with the apple slices.

Yield: 4 (2-tablespoons dip and 1/2-apple) servings

NUTRIENTS PER SERVING

Calories	147	Cholesterol	<1 mg	Fiber	3 g
Total Fat	5 g	Protein	5 g	Sodium	110 mg
Saturated Fat	1 g	Carbohydrates	22 g	Total Sugar	16 g

DIETARY EXCHANGES: 1 Medium Fat Protein, 1 Fruit
CARB CHOICES: 1

THERE IS NO SUCH THING IN ANYONE'S LIFE AS AN UNIMPORTANT DAY.

—ALEXANDER WOOLLCOTT

Garlic Herb Yogurt Cheese

2 cups plain nonfat yogurt
$1/4$ cup light mayonnaise
1 tablespoon dill weed, crushed
$3/4$ teaspoon garlic powder
$3/4$ teaspoon onion powder
$1/8$ teaspoon salt
$1/8$ teaspoon freshly ground pepper

Line a large strainer with a double thickness of 18×20-inch cheesecloth and place over a large bowl. Combine the yogurt, mayonnaise, dill weed, garlic powder, onion powder, salt and pepper in a bowl and mix well.

Spoon the yogurt mixture into the prepared strainer. Pull up the corners of the cheesecloth, twisting to enclose the yogurt completely. Chill for 24 hours or until all of the liquid has drained into the bowl and the yogurt is of a spreadable consistency. Place the cheese on a serving plate, discarding the cheesecloth and liquid. Serve with fresh vegetables and/or assorted party crackers.

Yield: 4 ($1/4$-cup) servings

NUTRIENTS PER SERVING

Calories	101	Cholesterol	3 mg	Fiber	<1 g
Total Fat	5 g	Protein	5 g	Sodium	249 mg
Saturated Fat	1 g	Carbohydrates	11 g	Total Sugar	7 g

DIETARY EXCHANGES: 1 Milk
CARB CHOICES: 1

Taco Cheese Spread

16 ounces light cream cheese, softened
1 cup plain nonfat yogurt, drained
2 envelopes taco seasoning mix
$1/2$ head lettuce, shredded
2 tomatoes, chopped
2 or 3 green onions, finely chopped
1 cup (4 ounces) shredded light
   Cheddar cheese

Beat the cream cheese, yogurt and seasoning mix in a bowl until blended. Spread the cream cheese mixture over the bottom of a pizza pan. Sprinkle with the lettuce, tomatoes, green onions and cheese. Serve with toasted bread rounds.

Yield: 20 servings

NUTRIENTS PER SERVING

Calories	67	Cholesterol	11 mg	Fiber	1 g
Total Fat	3 g	Protein	5 g	Sodium	282 mg
Saturated Fat	2 g	Carbohydrates	5 g	Total Sugar	2 g

DIETARY EXCHANGES: 1 Lean Meat
CARB CHOICES: 0

> NEVER LOOK DOWN ON ANYBODY UNLESS
> YOU'RE HELPING HIM UP.
>
> —JESSE JACKSON

Chicken Salad Ambrosia Spread

2 cups chopped cooked chicken breasts
1 (11-ounce) can mandarin oranges,
   drained and chopped
1 cup finely chopped celery
$1/2$ cup green grape halves
$1/2$ cup finely chopped pecans
$1/4$ cup light mayonnaise
$1/4$ cup light sour cream
$1 1/2$ teaspoons Italian salad dressing mix

Combine the chicken, mandarin oranges, celery, grapes and pecans in a bowl and mix well. Mix the mayonnaise, sour cream and salad dressing mix in a bowl and stir into the chicken mixture. Chill, covered, for 2 to 3 hours. Serve with assorted party crackers.

Yield: 10 servings

NUTRIENTS PER SERVING

Calories	144	Cholesterol	28 mg	Fiber	1 g
Total Fat	8 g	Protein	10 g	Sodium	181 mg
Saturated Fat	1 g	Carbohydrates	9 g	Total Sugar	7 g

DIETARY EXCHANGES: 1 Very Lean Protein, 1 Fruit, 1 Fat
CARB CHOICES: 1

Date Pecan Sandwiches

8 ounces light cream cheese, softened
2 tablespoons chopped dates
2 tablespoons chopped toasted pecans
1 tablespoon sour cream
$1/4$ teaspoon grated orange zest
8 slices whole wheat bread
1 cup finely shredded lettuce

Combine the cream cheese, dates, pecans, sour cream and orange zest in a bowl and mix well. Spread the cream cheese mixture evenly on one side of half of the bread slices and sprinkle evenly with the lettuce. Top with the remaining bread slices. Cut the sandwiches into quarters.

Yield: 16 (1-sandwich-quarter) servings

NUTRIENTS PER SERVING

Calories	67	Cholesterol	5 mg	Fiber	1 g
Total Fat	3 g	Protein	3 g	Sodium	127 mg
Saturated Fat	1 g	Carbohydrates	8 g	Total Sugar	2 g

DIETARY EXCHANGES: 1 Starch
CARB CHOICES: 1

> A TRUE FRIEND NEVER GETS IN YOUR WAY UNLESS
> YOU HAPPEN TO BE GOING DOWN.
>
> —ARNOLD H. GLASGOW

Salmon Salad Sandwiches

1 (16-ounce) can salmon, drained
2 hard-cooked eggs, chopped
$1/2$ cup light mayonnaise
$1/4$ cup finely chopped sweet pickle
1 tablespoon finely chopped onion
$1/2$ teaspoon prepared mustard
16 slices whole wheat bread
8 lettuce leaves

Discard the skin and bones from the salmon. Flake the salmon in a bowl and stir in the eggs, mayonnaise, pickle, onion and prepared mustard.

Spread the salmon mixture on one side of half of the bread slices and top each with one lettuce leaf. Top with the remaining bread slices and cut each sandwich diagonally into halves.

Yield: 16 ($1/2$-sandwich) servings

NUTRIENTS PER SERVING

Calories	146	Cholesterol	52 mg	Fiber	2 g
Total Fat	6 g	Protein	10 g	Sodium	354 mg
Saturated Fat	1 g	Carbohydrates	15 g	Total Sugar	2 g

DIETARY EXCHANGES: 1 Starch, 1 Lean Protein
CARB CHOICES: 1

Open-Face Hot Tuna Melts

6 light whole wheat English muffins,
   split into halves
2 (6-ounce) cans water-pack tuna, drained
3/4 cup chopped celery
1/3 cup finely chopped onion
1/3 cup mayonnaise-type salad dressing
1/8 teaspoon freshly ground pepper
12 slices sharp Cheddar cheese

Preheat the oven to 350 degrees. Arrange the muffins cut side up on a baking sheet. Mix the tuna, celery, onion, salad dressing and pepper in a bowl and spread over the muffins. Top each with one slice of cheese. Bake for 8 to 10 minutes or until brown and bubbly.

Yield: 12 servings

NUTRIENTS PER SERVING

Calories	229	Cholesterol	46 mg	Fiber	4 g
Total Fat	13 g	Protein	17 g	Sodium	440 mg
Saturated Fat	7 g	Carbohydrates	14 g	Total Sugar	1 g

DIETARY EXCHANGES: 1 Starch, 2 Lean Meat, 1 Fat
CARB CHOICES: 1

COURAGE IS NOT THE ABSENCE OF FEAR,
BUT RATHER THE JUDGMENT THAT SOMETHING ELSE
IS MORE IMPORTANT THAN FEAR.

—AMBROSE REDMOON

Waldorf Sandwiches

2 cups grated apples
1 tablespoon lemon juice
1 cup finely chopped celery
$1/2$ cup chopped pecans
$1/4$ cup light mayonnaise
10 slices cinnamon-raisin bread,
   crusts trimmed

Mix the apples, lemon juice, celery, pecans and mayonnaise in a bowl. Spread one side of each bread slice with the apple mixture. Cut the slices diagonally into halves.

Yield: 20 servings

NUTRIENTS PER SERVING

Calories	79	Cholesterol	1 mg	Fiber	1 g
Total Fat	4 g	Protein	2 g	Sodium	81 mg
Saturated Fat	<1 g	Carbohydrates	10 g	Total Sugar	5 g

DIETARY EXCHANGES: 1 Fruit
CARB CHOICES: 1

MY MOST BRILLIANT ACHIEVEMENT WAS MY ABILITY TO
BE ABLE TO PERSUADE MY WIFE TO MARRY ME.

—WINSTON CHURCHILL

Snack Oat Cookies

PHOTOGRAPH FOR THIS RECIPE APPEARS ON PAGE 14.

4 cups all-purpose flour
$2^{1}/_{2}$ cups rolled oats
$1^{1}/_{2}$ cups Splenda
1 tablespoon baking soda
1 teaspoon baking powder
1 teaspoon salt
$1^{1}/_{2}$ teaspoons ground cinnamon
$1/_{2}$ cup unsweetened applesauce

$1/_{2}$ cup baby food prunes
5 egg whites, lightly beaten
$1/_{2}$ to 1 cup water
$1^{1}/_{2}$ teaspoons vanilla extract
$3/_{4}$ cup raisins
$1/_{2}$ cup (3 ounces) miniature
   chocolate chips

Preheat the oven to 350 degrees. Combine the flour, oats, artificial sweetener, baking soda, baking powder, salt and cinnamon in a bowl and mix well. Make a well in the center of the flour mixture and add the applesauce, prunes, egg whites, water and vanilla to the well. Stir just until moistened and fold in the raisins and chocolate chips.

Shape the dough with moist hands into balls the size of a golf ball. Arrange the balls on a greased cookie sheet and flatten until $1/_{2}$ inch thick. Bake for 8 to 10 minutes for a chewy cookie or 10 to 12 minutes for a crisp cookie. Cool on the cookie sheet for 2 minutes and remove to a wire rack to cool completely. Serve with a glass of skim milk. Store in an airtight container.

Yield: 14 cookies

NUTRIENTS PER COOKIE

Calories	295	Cholesterol	0 mg	Fiber	3 g
Total Fat	4 g	Protein	8 g	Sodium	493 mg
Saturated Fat	2 g	Carbohydrates	58 g	Total Sugar	8 g

DIETARY EXCHANGES: 2 Starch, 1 Other Carbohydrate/Sugar, 1 Fruit
CARB CHOICES: 4

Bacon and Cheese Tomato Cups

1 (10-count) can flaky biscuits
8 slices turkey bacon, crisp-cooked and crumbled
3 ounces Swiss cheese, shredded
1 tomato, peeled and chopped
$1/2$ small onion, finely chopped
1 teaspoon basil
$1/2$ cup light mayonnaise

Preheat the oven to 375 degrees. Separate each biscuit into three layers. Press each biscuit layer into a miniature muffin cup. Combine the bacon, cheese, tomato, onion and basil in a bowl and mix well. Fold in the mayonnaise.

Fill each prepared muffin cup with an equal portion of the bacon mixture. Bake for 10 to 12 minutes or until brown. You may substitute $1/2$ to $3/4$ cup commercially prepared salsa for the tomato and onion.

Yield: 30 cups

NUTRIENTS PER CUP

Calories	67	Cholesterol	7 mg	Fiber	<1 g
Total Fat	4 g	Protein	2 g	Sodium	205 mg
Saturated Fat	1 g	Carbohydrates	5 g	Total Sugar	1 g

DIETARY EXCHANGES: 1 Vegetable, 1 Fat,
CARB CHOICES: 0

WHEN YOU REACH THE END OF YOUR ROPE,
TIE A KNOT IN IT AND HANG ON.

—THOMAS JEFFERSON

Honey-Baked Chicken Wings

18 chicken wings (about 3 pounds)
1 1/2 cups dry bread crumbs
1/4 cup sesame seeds
1 1/4 teaspoons salt
3/4 teaspoon ground ginger
3/4 teaspoon paprika
1/8 teaspoon red pepper
1 cup plain fat-free yogurt
2 tablespoons honey
6 tablespoons margarine, melted

Preheat the oven to 425 degrees. Cut each wing into three joints, discarding the tips. Mix the bread crumbs, sesame seeds, salt, ginger, paprika and red pepper in a shallow dish. Mix the yogurt and honey in a bowl. Dip the chicken wings in the yogurt mixture and coat with the bread crumb mixture.

Arrange the coated chicken wings on a rack in a large roasting pan and drizzle with 3 tablespoons of the margarine. Bake for 15 minutes and drizzle with the remaining 3 tablespoons margarine. Bake for 15 minutes longer or until brown and tender.

Yield: 36 servings

NUTRIENTS PER SERVING

Calories	88	Cholesterol	12 mg	Fiber	1 g
Total Fat	5 g	Protein	5 g	Sodium	152 mg
Saturated Fat	1 g	Carbohydrates	5 g	Total Sugar	2 g

DIETARY EXCHANGES: 1 Medium Fat Protein
CARB CHOICES: 0

Parmesan Chicken Strips

8 ounces boneless skinless chicken breasts
$1/4$ cup (1 ounce) grated fat-free
   Parmesan cheese
$1/4$ teaspoon chili powder or Hungarian paprika, or to taste
$1/2$ teaspoon oregano
$1/2$ teaspoon basil
$1/8$ teaspoon garlic powder
Salt and freshly ground pepper to taste
1 egg, beaten

Preheat the oven to 350 degrees. Cut the chicken into 1-inch strips. Mix the cheese, chili powder, oregano, basil, garlic powder, salt and pepper in a shallow dish. Dip the chicken in the egg and coat with the cheese mixture.

Arrange the coated chicken strips on a baking sheet sprayed with nonstick cooking spray. Bake for 18 to 20 minutes or until the chicken is cooked through and light brown, turning once. Serve with fat-free ranch salad dressing, if desired.

Yield: 10 servings

NUTRIENTS PER SERVING

Calories	38	Cholesterol	34 mg	Fiber	<1 g
Total Fat	1 g	Protein	6 g	Sodium	58 mg
Saturated Fat	<1 g	Carbohydrates	<1 g	Total Sugar	<1 g

DIETARY EXCHANGES: 1 Very Lean Protein
CARB CHOICES: 0

> NO ACT OF KINDNESS, HOWEVER SMALL, IS EVER WASTED.
>
> —AESOP

Chicken Sesame Nibbles

8 ounces light cream cheese, softened
$1/2$ teaspoon lemon juice
1 teaspoon Italian seasoning
$1/4$ teaspoon onion powder
1 cup finely chopped cooked chicken breast
$1/3$ cup finely chopped celery
2 (8-count) cans crescent rolls
1 egg white, beaten
1 tablespoon sesame seeds

Preheat the oven to 375 degrees. Beat the cream cheese, lemon juice, Italian seasoning and onion powder in a mixing bowl until blended. Stir in the chicken and celery. Separate the roll dough into eight rectangles and press the perforations to seal. Spread the chicken mixture evenly over the rectangles, leaving a $1/2$-inch border.

Roll each rectangle from the long side to enclose the filling. Brush with the egg white and sprinkle with the sesame seeds. Cut each roll into five portions and arrange seam side down on a baking sheet sprayed with nonstick cooking spray. Bake for 12 minutes or until golden brown.

Yield: 40 chicken nibbles

NUTRIENTS PER NIBBLE

Calories	60	Cholesterol	5 mg	Fiber	<1 g
Total Fat	3 g	Protein	3 g	Sodium	115 mg
Saturated Fat	1 g	Carbohydrates	5 g	Total Sugar	1 g

DIETARY EXCHANGES: 1 Fat
CARB CHOICES: 0

Chile Cheese Pick-Ups

$1/2$ cup all-purpose flour
1 teaspoon baking powder
$1/2$ teaspoon salt
8 eggs
2 cups nonfat cottage cheese
4 ounces Monterey Jack cheese, shredded
$1/4$ cup ($1/2$ stick) butter, melted
1 (4-ounce) can chopped green chiles

Preheat the oven to 350 degrees. Mix the flour, baking powder and salt in a bowl. Whisk the eggs in a bowl until blended. Stir in the flour mixture, cottage cheese, Monterey Jack cheese, butter and green chiles.

Pour the egg mixture into a medium baking dish sprayed with nonstick cooking spray. Bake for 40 minutes or until puffed and firm to the touch. Cool slightly and cut into squares. Serve warm.

Yield: 24 (1-square) servings

NUTRIENTS PER SERVING

Calories	84	Cholesterol	81 mg	Fiber	<1 g
Total Fat	5 g	Protein	6 g	Sodium	263 mg
Saturated Fat	3 g	Carbohydrates	3 g	Total Sugar	1 g

DIETARY EXCHANGES: 1 Medium Fat Protein
CARB CHOICES: 0

PUT ALL EXCUSES ASIDE AND REMEMBER THIS:
YOU ARE CAPABLE.

—ZIG ZIGLAR

Cheesy Spinach Rolls

1 (1-pound) loaf frozen
  bread dough
1 (10-ounce) package frozen
  chopped spinach, thawed
  and drained

4 ounces feta cheese, crumbled
4 green onions, thinly sliced
1 tablespoon Greek seasoning

Thaw the bread dough using the package directions. Spray fifteen muffin cups with nonstick cooking spray. Roll the dough into a 9×15-inch rectangle on a lightly floured surface. If the dough is too difficult to roll, cover with plastic wrap and let rest for 5 minutes. Position the dough so the long side runs parallel to the edge of the work surface.

Press the excess moisture from the spinach. Mix the spinach with the cheese, green onions and Greek seasoning in a bowl. Spread the spinach mixture over the dough to within 1 inch of the long sides. Starting at the long side, roll to enclose the filling and pinch the seam to seal. Arrange the roll seam side down and cut into fifteen 1-inch slices using a serrated knife. Arrange the slices cut side up in the prepared muffin cups. Let stand, covered with plastic wrap, in a warm place for 30 minutes or until the slices are slightly puffy.

Preheat the oven to 375 degrees. Bake for 20 to 25 minutes or until golden brown. Serve warm or at room temperature. The rolls may be stored in an airtight container in the refrigerator for up to 2 days.

Yield: 15 rolls

NUTRIENTS PER ROLL

Calories	109	Cholesterol	7 mg	Fiber	1 g
Total Fat	3 g	Protein	5 g	Sodium	464 mg
Saturated Fat	1 g	Carbohydrates	17 g	Total Sugar	2 g

DIETARY EXCHANGES: 1 Starch
CARB CHOICES: 1

Baked Zucchini Bites

1 cup shredded zucchini, drained
$1/4$ cup light mayonnaise
$1/4$ cup plain low-fat yogurt
2 tablespoons grated Parmesan cheese
2 green onions, thinly sliced
$1/2$ teaspoon Worcestershire sauce
$1/8$ teaspoon hot pepper sauce
1 small garlic clove, minced
24 slices party rye bread

Preheat the oven to 375 degrees. Squeeze the excess moisture from the zucchini and mix with the mayonnaise, yogurt, cheese, green onions, Worcestershire sauce, hot sauce and garlic in a bowl.

Spread 1 rounded teaspoonful of the zucchini mixture on each bread slice. Arrange the slices on a baking sheet and bake for 12 minutes or until brown and bubbly.

Yield: 24 bites

NUTRIENTS PER BITE

Calories	38	Cholesterol	1 mg	Fiber	1 g
Total Fat	1 g	Protein	1 g	Sodium	117 mg
Saturated Fat	<1 g	Carbohydrates	6 g	Total Sugar	1 g

DIETARY EXCHANGES: 1 Vegetable
CARB CHOICES: 0

THE JOURNEY IS THE REWARD.

—CHINESE PROVERB

Tater-Dipped Veggies

1 cup instant potato flakes
$1/3$ cup grated Parmesan cheese
$1/4$ teaspoon celery powder
$1/8$ to $1/4$ teaspoon garlic powder
$1/4$ cup reduced-calorie margarine, melted
3 egg whites
4 cups assorted fresh vegetable chunks

Preheat the oven to 400 degrees. Combine the potato flakes, cheese, celery powder and garlic powder in a bowl and mix well. Stir in the margarine. Whisk the egg whites in a bowl until foamy.

Dip the vegetables in the egg whites and then in the potato flake mixture. Arrange the coated vegetables on a baking sheet sprayed with nonstick cooking spray and bake for 15 to 20 minutes or until light brown. Serve immediately.

Yield: 8 servings

NUTRIENTS PER SERVING

Calories	84	Cholesterol	3 mg	Fiber	2 g
Total Fat	4 g	Protein	4 g	Sodium	165 mg
Saturated Fat	1 g	Carbohydrates	9 g	Total Sugar	2 g

DIETARY EXCHANGES: 1 Starch
CARB CHOICES: 1

Cold Veggie Pizza

2 cups reduced-fat baking mix
2/3 cup skim milk
6 ounces fat-free mozzarella cheese, shredded
4 ounces fat-free cream cheese, softened
1/4 cup fat-free mayonnaise-type salad dressing
1/2 cup fat-free sour cream
1 envelope ranch salad dressing mix
1 teaspoon garlic powder (optional)
1 cup chopped fresh broccoli
1 cup chopped fresh cauliflower

Preheat the oven to 350 degrees. Mix the baking mix and skim milk in a bowl with a fork until the mixture forms a ball. Press the dough over the bottom and up the side of a pizza pan. Bake for 8 to 10 minutes. Let stand until cool.

Beat the mozzarella cheese, cream cheese, salad dressing, sour cream, salad dressing mix and garlic powder in a bowl until blended, scraping the bowl occasionally. Spread the cheese mixture over the baked layer and sprinkle with the broccoli and cauliflower. Chill, covered, until serving time. Cut into wedges.

Yield: 12 (1-wedge) servings

NUTRIENTS PER SERVING

Calories	136	Cholesterol	4 mg	Fiber	1 g
Total Fat	2 g	Protein	9 g	Sodium	635 mg
Saturated Fat	<1 g	Carbohydrates	21 g	Total Sugar	3 g

DIETARY EXCHANGES:1 Bread, 1 Vegetable
CARB CHOICES: 1

Seasoning Shake

6 tablespoons onion powder
3 tablespoons paprika
3 tablespoons poultry seasoning
2 tablespoons dry mustard
1 tablespoon garlic powder
2 teaspoons oregano
2 teaspoons freshly ground pepper
1 teaspoon chili powder

Mix the onion powder, paprika, poultry seasoning, dry mustard, garlic powder, oregano, pepper and chili powder in a bowl. Store in a jar with a tight-fitting lid in a cool environment. Use as a seasoning on meat, poultry, seafood or vegetables.

Reduce the intake of sodium in recipes by substituting Seasoning Shake for the salt.

Yield: 50 teaspoons

NUTRIENTS PER TEASPOON

Calories	8	Cholesterol	0 mg	Fiber	<1 g
Total Fat	<1 g	Protein	<1 g	Sodium	2 mg
Saturated Fat	<1 g	Carbohydrates	1 g	Total Sugar	<1 g

DIETARY EXCHANGES: Free
CARB CHOICES: 0

> TREAT YOUR FRIENDS AS YOU DO YOUR PICTURES,
> AND PLACE THEM IN THEIR BEST LIGHT.
>
> —JENNIE JEROME CHURCHILL

Entrées Contents

Entrées

Salsa-Topped
Tilapia
page 78

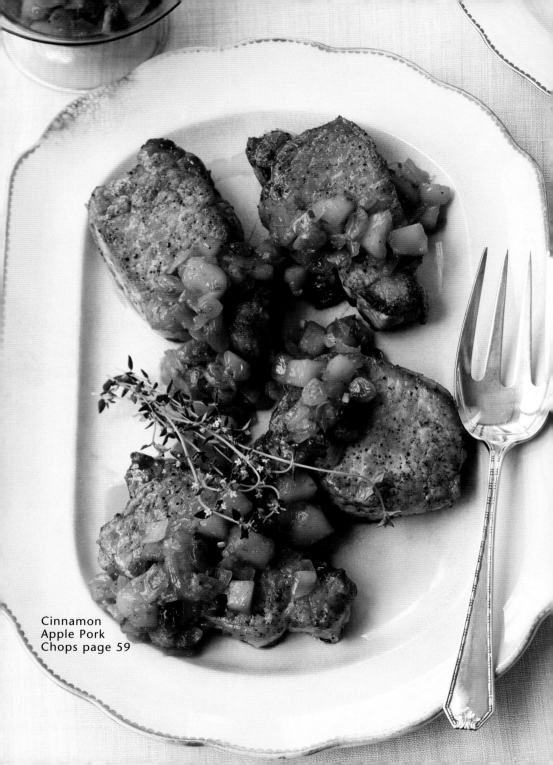

Cinnamon
Apple Pork
Chops page 59

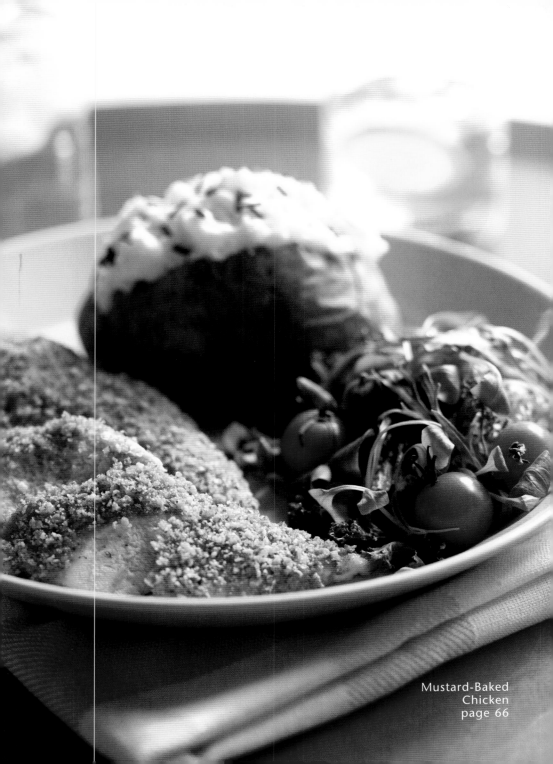

Mustard-Baked
Chicken
page 66

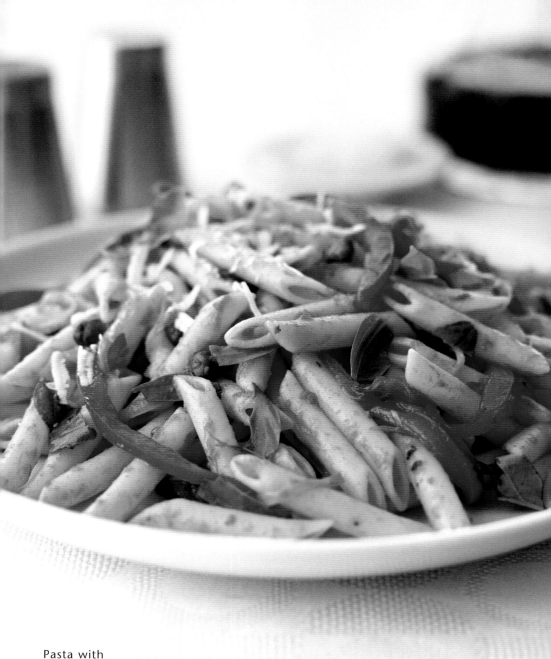

Pasta with
Red Pepper Sauce
page 82

Lemon Herb Chuck Roast

PHOTOGRAPH FOR THIS RECIPE APPEARS ON PAGE 3.

2 teaspoons lemon pepper
1 teaspoon basil
2 garlic cloves, crushed
1 (3-pound) boneless beef
  chuck roast, trimmed
1 tablespoon olive oil
1 cup water

1 pound small red potatoes,
  cut into halves
2 cups baby carrots
1 onion, cut into 6 wedges
2 tablespoons cornstarch
2 tablespoons water
1/2 teaspoon basil

Mix the lemon pepper, 1 teaspoon basil and the garlic in a bowl and rub the garlic mixture over the surface of the roast. Heat the olive oil in a Dutch oven over medium-high heat until hot. Add the roast to the hot oil and cook until brown on all sides, turning several times; drain. Add 1 cup water and simmer, covered, for 2 hours.

Add the potatoes, carrots and onion and simmer, covered, for 40 to 45 minutes or until the vegetables are tender and the roast is the desired degree of doneness. Remove the roast and vegetables to a heated platter, reserving the pan drippings.

Skim the fat from the drippings and stir in a mixture of the cornstarch and 2 tablespoons water. Mix in 1/2 teaspoon basil and bring to a boil. Cook until thickened, stirring constantly. Serve the gravy with the roast and vegetables.

Yield: 6 servings

NUTRIENTS PER SERVING

Calories	485	Cholesterol	156 mg	Fiber	3 g
Total Fat	22 g	Protein	48 g	Sodium	284 mg
Saturated Fat	8 g	Carbohydrates	21 g	Total Sugar	4 g

DIETARY EXCHANGES: 1 Starch, 6 Lean Meat, 1 Vegetable, 1 Fat
CARB CHOICES: 1

Moroccan Pot Roast

1 cup dried apricots
1 cup water
1 (5-pound) boneless beef top round or bottom round roast, trimmed
2 teaspoons salt
$1/4$ teaspoon freshly ground pepper

$1/2$ teaspoon ground ginger
1 tablespoon canola oil
2 cups sliced fresh mushrooms
$1^{1}/2$ cups chopped onions
1 (6-ounce) can pitted black olives, drained
$1/2$ cup water or red wine
2 garlic cloves, finely chopped

Plump the apricots in 1 cup water in a bowl and drain. Rub the surface of the roast with a mixture of the salt, pepper and ginger. Heat the canola oil in a large skillet and add the roast to the hot oil. Cook until brown on all sides, turning occasionally. Drain and place the roast in a slow cooker.

Add the apricots, mushrooms, onions, olives, $1/2$ cup water and the garlic to the slow cooker and cook, covered, on Low for 8 hours. You may bake in a 325-degree oven for 3 hours.

Yield: 12 servings

NUTRIENTS PER SERVING

Calories	314	Cholesterol	113 mg	Fiber	2 g
Total Fat	12 g	Protein	38 g	Sodium	573 mg
Saturated Fat	3 g	Carbohydrates	12 g	Total Sugar	7 g

DIETARY EXCHANGES: 5 Lean Meat, 2 Vegetable
CARB CHOICES: 1

I'M NOT RUSHING INTO BEING IN LOVE.
I'M FINDING FOURTH GRADE HARD ENOUGH.

—REGINA, AGE 10

Cranberry-Glazed Pot Roast

1 teaspoon canola oil
1 (4-pound) boneless top sirloin
  roast, trimmed
1 (10-ounce) can beef broth
$3/4$ cup whole cranberry sauce
$1/2$ cup ketchup
$1/2$ envelope dry onion soup mix

2 garlic cloves, minced
1 teaspoon dry mustard
$1/2$ teaspoon marjoram
$1/4$ teaspoon freshly
  ground pepper
10 potatoes, quartered
5 large carrots, quartered

Preheat the oven to 350 degrees. Heat the canola oil in a large skillet and add the roast. Cook until brown on all sides, turning occasionally. Remove the roast to a roasting pan. Whisk the broth, cranberry sauce, ketchup, soup mix, garlic, dry mustard, marjoram and pepper in a bowl and pour over the roast.

Bake, covered, for 2 hours, basting occasionally with the pan juices. Add the potatoes and carrots to the roasting pan and spoon the pan juices over the vegetables. Bake for 1 hour longer. Slice the roast as desired and arrange on a serving platter surrounded by the vegetables. Serve with the pan juices.

Yield: 10 servings

NUTRIENTS PER SERVING

Calories	322	Cholesterol	67 mg	Fiber	5 g
Total Fat	8 g	Protein	40 g	Sodium	370 mg
Saturated Fat	3 g	Carbohydrates	22 g	Total Sugar	12 g

DIETARY EXCHANGES: 1 Starch, 4 Lean Meat, 1 Vegetable
CARB CHOICES: 1

Sirloin Steak with Creamy Mushroom Sauce

1 (2-pound) sirloin steak,
  2 inches thick
1 teaspoon coarsely
  ground pepper
3 cups sliced fresh mushrooms
1 cup sliced green onions
2 teaspoons dry mustard

2 tablespoons butter
1 tablespoon
  Worcestershire sauce
1 tablespoon lemon juice
1/4 cup chopped fresh parsley
3/4 cup evaporated skim milk

Preheat the broiler. Rub the steak with the pepper and arrange on a broiler rack in a broiler pan. Broil for 10 minutes per side for medium or until the desired degree of doneness, turning once. Cover to keep warm.

Sauté the mushrooms, green onions and dry mustard in the butter in a nonstick skillet until the mushrooms are tender. Stir in the Worcestershire sauce, lemon juice and parsley. Cook for 1 minute and stir in the evaporated skim milk.

Cook until heated through and of a sauce consistency, stirring constantly; do not boil. Slice the steak as desired and serve with the mushroom sauce.

Yield: 6 servings

NUTRIENTS PER SERVING

Calories	261	Cholesterol	67 mg	Fiber	1 g
Total Fat	10 g	Protein	34 g	Sodium	159 mg
Saturated Fat	5 g	Carbohydrates	7 g	Total Sugar	5 g

DIETARY EXCHANGES: 4 Lean Meat, 1 Vegetable
CARB CHOICES: 1/2

LOVE IS WHAT MAKES YOU SMILE WHEN YOU'RE TIRED.

Manicotti

1 pound lean ground beef
$1/4$ cup chopped onion
3 slices whole wheat bread, torn
$1/2$ cup skim milk
1 egg, beaten
Salt and freshly ground pepper
   to taste
8 ounces manicotti shells
4 cups water
1 (4-ounce) can mushrooms

1 (15-ounce) can no-added-salt
   tomato sauce
1 (12-ounce) can tomato paste
$1/4$ cup chopped onion
$1/4$ teaspoon garlic powder
$1/4$ teaspoon freshly
   ground pepper
1 cup (4 ounces) shredded
   mozzarella cheese

Preheat the oven to 375 degrees. Brown the ground beef with $1/4$ cup onion in a skillet, stirring until the ground beef is crumbly; drain. Combine the ground beef mixture, bread, skim milk, egg, salt and pepper in a bowl and mix well. Stuff the ground beef mixture into the manicotti shells. Place the stuffed shells in a single layer in a 9×13-inch baking pan sprayed with nonstick cooking spray.

Mix the water, undrained mushrooms, tomato sauce, tomato paste, $1/4$ cup onion, the garlic powder and $1/4$ teaspoon pepper in a saucepan and simmer for 5 minutes, stirring occasionally. Pour the mushroom mixture over the manicotti and sprinkle with the cheese. Bake, covered, for $1 1/2$ hours.

Yield: 6 servings

NUTRIENTS PER SERVING

Calories	475	Cholesterol	98 mg	Fiber	6 g
Total Fat	16 g	Protein	31 g	Sodium	789 mg
Saturated Fat	7 g	Carbohydrates	54 g	Total Sugar	15 g

DIETARY EXCHANGES: 3 Starch, 3 Lean Meat, 1 Vegetable, 1 Fat
CARB CHOICES: 3

Shepherd's Pie

1 pound extra-lean ground beef (93/7)
$1/2$ cup chopped onion
1 envelope brown gravy mix
1 cup water
1 (10-ounce) package frozen peas and carrots
3 cups mashed potatoes
Shredded Cheddar cheese (optional)

Brown the ground beef with the onion in a skillet, stirring until the ground beef is crumbly; drain. Whisk the gravy mix and water in a bowl until blended and stir the gravy into the ground beef mixture. Cook until thickened, stirring frequently. Stir in the peas and carrots and simmer, covered, for 5 minutes.

Preheat the oven to 400 degrees. Spoon the ground beef mixture into a $1^{1/2}$-quart baking dish and spread with the mashed potatoes. Sprinkle with cheese and bake for 20 minutes or until the mashed potatoes are brown.

Yield: 6 (1-cup) servings

NUTRIENTS PER SERVING

Calories	277	Cholesterol	42 mg	Fiber	3 g
Total Fat	10 g	Protein	21 g	Sodium	610 mg
Saturated Fat	5 g	Carbohydrates	27 g	Total Sugar	2 g

DIETARY EXCHANGES: 1 Starch, 2 Lean Meat, 1 Fat
CARB CHOICES: 1

Cinnamon Apple Pork Chops

PHOTOGRAPH FOR THIS RECIPE APPEARS ON PAGE 50.

4 ($3^1/2$-ounce) loin pork chops
$1/4$ cup all-purpose flour
1 teaspoon chopped fresh
   parsley, or 1 tablespoon
   parsley flakes
$1/4$ teaspoon salt

$2/3$ cup water
2 cups chopped unpeeled apples
3 tablespoons brown sugar
$1/4$ teaspoon ground cinnamon
Sprigs of thyme for garnish

Preheat the oven to 325 degrees. Brown the pork chops on both sides in a skillet and arrange in a single layer in a baking dish. Sprinkle with the flour, parsley and salt. Drizzle with $1/3$ cup of the water.

Bake, covered with foil, for 30 minutes. Toss the apples with the brown sugar and cinnamon in a bowl until coated and spoon the apple mixture over the pork chops. Drizzle with the remaining $1/3$ cup water and bake, covered, for 20 minutes. Remove the foil and bake for 10 minutes longer. Garnish with sprigs of thyme.

Yield: 4 servings

NUTRIENTS PER SERVING

Calories	246	Cholesterol	63 mg	Fiber	2 g
Total Fat	6 g	Protein	23 g	Sodium	196 mg
Saturated Fat	2 g	Carbohydrates	24 g	Total Sugar	16 g

DIETARY EXCHANGES: 3 Lean Meat, 1 Fruit, 1 Vegetable
CARB CHOICES: 1

THERE ARE NO GREAT THINGS, ONLY SMALL THINGS
WITH GREAT LOVE. HAPPY ARE THOSE.

—MOTHER TERESA

Pork Chops Florentine

1/2 cup thawed frozen
  chopped spinach
1 tablespoon butter
4 (3 1/2-ounce) boneless pork
  chops, 3/4 inch thick
1 cup finely chopped
  fresh mushrooms

1/3 cup minced red onion
1 egg, lightly beaten
1/2 teaspoon salt
1/8 teaspoon freshly
  ground pepper
3 tablespoons shredded
  Cheddar cheese

Preheat the oven to 350 degrees. Press the excess moisture from the spinach. Melt the butter in a nonstick skillet and add the pork chops. Sear the pork chops in the butter to seal in the juices. Remove the pork chops to a baking dish, reserving the pan drippings. Sauté the mushrooms in the pan drippings until the mushrooms are tender and most of the moisture has evaporated. Let stand until cool.

Combine the mushrooms, spinach, onion, egg, salt and pepper in a bowl and mix well. Spoon the mushroom mixture over the pork chops and bake for 30 minutes. Sprinkle with the cheese and bake for 10 minutes longer or until the chops are cooked through and the juices run clear when pierced with a fork.

Yield: 4 servings

NUTRIENTS PER SERVING

Calories	234	Cholesterol	129 mg	Fiber	1 g
Total Fat	12 g	Protein	26 g	Sodium	469 mg
Saturated Fat	6 g	Carbohydrates	3 g	Total Sugar	1 g

DIETARY EXCHANGES: 4 Lean Meat
CARB CHOICES: 0

Oven-Fried Pork Chops

1 egg white
2 tablespoons unsweetened
  pineapple juice
1 tablespoon light soy sauce
$1/4$ teaspoon ground ginger
$1/8$ teaspoon garlic powder

$1/3$ cup plain bread crumbs
$1/2$ teaspoon Italian seasoning
$1/4$ teaspoon paprika
Garlic powder to taste
4 (5-ounce) center-cut
  pork chops

Preheat the oven to 350 degrees. Whisk the egg white, pineapple juice, soy sauce, ginger and $1/8$ teaspoon garlic powder in a bowl until blended. Mix the bread crumbs, Italian seasoning, paprika and garlic powder to taste in a shallow dish.

Dip the pork chops in the egg white mixture and coat with the bread crumb mixture. Arrange the pork chops in a single layer on a rack sprayed with nonstick cooking spray in a baking pan. Bake for 50 minutes, turning halfway through the baking process.

Yield: 4 servings

NUTRIENTS PER SERVING

Calories	242	Cholesterol	83 mg	Fiber	<1 g
Total Fat	9 g	Protein	31 g	Sodium	365 mg
Saturated Fat	3 g	Carbohydrates	8 g	Total Sugar	1 g

DIETARY EXCHANGES: 4 Lean Protein, 1 Vegetable
CARB CHOICES: $1/2$

THERE ARE ONLY TWO WAYS TO LIVE YOUR LIFE. ONE IS AS THOUGH NOTHING IS A MIRACLE. THE OTHER IS AS IF EVERYTHING IS.

—ALBERT EINSTEIN

Pork Chop Stew

4 potatoes, peeled
   and quartered
4 large carrots, peeled and
   cut into chunks
1 onion, chopped
1 green bell pepper,
   cut into strips

$1/2$ teaspoon oregano
$1/2$ teaspoon curry powder
$1/2$ teaspoon sage
4 ($3^1/2$-ounce) pork chops
Salt and freshly ground pepper
   to taste

Preheat the oven to 350 degrees. Toss the potatoes, carrots, onion, bell pepper, oregano, curry powder and sage in a 9×13-inch baking dish. Add just enough water to cover the vegetables. Arrange the pork chops over the vegetables and sprinkle with salt and pepper.

Bake, covered with foil, for $1^1/2$ hours or until the pork chops are cooked through, turning once.

Yield: 4 servings

NUTRIENTS PER SERVING

Calories	356	Cholesterol	63 mg	Fiber	6 g
Total Fat	7 g	Protein	27 g	Sodium	109 mg
Saturated Fat	2 g	Carbohydrates	47 g	Total Sugar	8 g

DIETARY EXCHANGES: 2 Starch, 3 Lean Meat, 2 Vegetable
CARB CHOICES: 3

PEOPLE ARE LIKE STAINED-GLASS WINDOWS. THEY
SPARKLE AND SHINE WHEN THE SUN IS OUT, BUT WHEN THE
DARKNESS SETS IN, THEIR TRUE BEAUTY IS REVEALED
ONLY IF THERE IS A LIGHT FROM WITHIN.

—ELIZABETH KUBLER ROSS

Citrus-Poached Chicken Breasts

$1^{1}/_{2}$ cups orange juice
$1^{1}/_{4}$ cups canned chicken broth
3 large scallions, chopped
6 (5-ounce) boneless skinless chicken breasts
$1/4$ cup all-purpose flour
3 bunches watercress
Sections of 1 large orange, cut into halves

Combine the orange juice, broth and scallions in a large saucepan and simmer for 2 minutes, stirring occasionally. Add the chicken to the hot mixture and simmer, loosely covered, for 20 minutes or until the chicken is cooked through. Remove the chicken to a serving platter using a slotted spoon, reserving the poaching liquid. Cover loosely to keep warm.

Mix $1/4$ cup of the reserved poaching liquid with the flour in a bowl until blended. Bring the remaining poaching liquid to a boil and whisk in the flour mixture. Cook until thickened, whisking constantly.

Arrange equal amounts of the watercress on each of six dinner plates. Arrange one chicken breast on each prepared plate and drizzle with equal amounts of the sauce. Top with the orange sections.

Yield: 6 servings

NUTRIENTS PER SERVING

Calories	222	Cholesterol	79 mg	Fiber	1 g
Total Fat	4 g	Protein	31 g	Sodium	282 mg
Saturated Fat	1 g	Carbohydrates	15 g	Total Sugar	9 g

DIETARY EXCHANGES: 1 Starch, 4 Very Lean Protein
CARB CHOICES: 1

Chicken Parmesan

$1/3$ cup water
$1/4$ cup (1 ounce) grated
  Parmesan cheese
$1/4$ cup bread crumbs
$1/4$ teaspoon garlic powder
1 tablespoon parsley flakes
$1/4$ teaspoon freshly
  ground pepper

$1/4$ teaspoon paprika
$1/8$ teaspoon thyme
4 (5-ounce) boneless skinless
  chicken breasts
1 tablespoon canola oil
1 tablespoon margarine, melted
$1/3$ cup Marsala wine

Preheat the oven to 350 degrees. Spray a baking pan with nonstick cooking spray and add the water. Toss the cheese, bread crumbs, garlic powder, parsley flakes, pepper, paprika and thyme in a shallow dish. Coat the chicken with the cheese mixture and arrange in the prepared pan. Drizzle with the canola oil and margarine.

Bake for 30 minutes and drizzle with the wine. Reduce the oven temperature to 325 degrees and bake, covered with foil, for 10 minutes. Remove the foil and bake for 10 minutes longer or until the chicken is tender and cooked through.

Yield: 4 servings

NUTRIENTS PER SERVING

Calories	289	Cholesterol	83 mg	Fiber	<1 g
Total Fat	11 g	Protein	32 g	Sodium	230 mg
Saturated Fat	3 g	Carbohydrates	8 g	Total Sugar	2 g

DIETARY EXCHANGES: $1/2$ Other Carbohydrate/Sugar, 4 Lean Protein
CARB CHOICES: $1/2$

> WHETHER YOU THINK YOU CAN OR WHETHER YOU
> THINK YOU CAN'T, YOU'RE RIGHT!
>
> —HENRY FORD

Chicken Piccata

2 egg whites
6 (5-ounce) boneless skinless
  chicken breasts
$1/3$ cup all-purpose flour
2 tablespoons olive oil
$1/2$ onion, chopped
2 green onions, chopped
$1/2$ green bell pepper, chopped
Chopped fresh parsley to taste

1 tablespoon olive oil
1 tablespoon all-purpose flour
$1/2$ cup canned fat-free
  chicken broth
$1/3$ cup white wine or apple juice
1 (8-ounce) can no-added-salt
  tomato sauce
Salt and freshly ground pepper
  to taste

Beat the egg whites in a mixing bowl just until foamy. Pound the chicken between sheets of waxed paper until flattened. Coat the chicken with $1/3$ cup flour and dip in the egg whites. Sauté in 2 tablespoons olive oil in a skillet until brown on both sides and cooked through. Remove the chicken to a heated platter using a slotted spoon and cover to keep warm.

Sauté the onion, green onions, bell pepper and parsley in 1 tablespoon olive oil in a nonstick skillet until the onion is tender. Sprinkle with 1 tablespoon flour and stir in the broth, wine and tomato sauce. Season to taste with salt and pepper. Cook until of the desired consistency, stirring constantly. Add the chicken and cook until heated through, stirring occasionally.

Yield: 6 servings

NUTRIENTS PER SERVING

Calories	272	Cholesterol	73 mg	Fiber	1 g
Total Fat	10 g	Protein	30 g	Sodium	121 mg
Saturated Fat	2 g	Carbohydrates	11 g	Total Sugar	3 g

DIETARY EXCHANGES: 1 Starch, 4 Very Lean Meat, 1 Fat
CARB CHOICES: 1

Mustard-Baked Chicken

PHOTOGRAPH FOR THIS RECIPE APPEARS ON PAGE 51.

6 (5-ounce) chicken breasts, skinned
Salt and freshly ground pepper to taste
$1/2$ cup prepared mustard
2 tablespoons light brown sugar
$1^1/2$ cups plain dry bread crumbs

Preheat the oven to 400 degrees. Season the chicken with salt and pepper. Arrange the chicken on a rack sprayed with nonstick cooking spray in a roasting pan. Roast for 10 to 15 minutes or until light brown, turning occasionally. Maintain the oven temperature.

Mix the prepared mustard and brown sugar in a bowl. Spread the mustard mixture over the chicken and coat with the bread crumbs. Bake for 20 minutes and turn the chicken. Bake for 10 to 20 minutes longer or until the chicken is cooked through and golden brown. Serve with mixed salad greens and a baked potato.

Yield: 6 servings

NUTRIENTS PER SERVING

Calories	294	Cholesterol	78 mg	Fiber	2 g
Total Fat	6 g	Protein	33 g	Sodium	529 mg
Saturated Fat	1 g	Carbohydrates	25 g	Total Sugar	7 g

DIETARY EXCHANGES: 2 Starch, 4 Very Lean Protein
CARB CHOICES: 2

Orange Thyme Chicken

4 (5-ounce) boneless skinless chicken breasts
$1/2$ cup fresh orange juice
2 tablespoons olive oil
2 tablespoons honey
1 tablespoon fresh thyme leaves, or
   1 teaspoon dried thyme
Salt and freshly ground pepper to taste

Arrange the chicken in a single layer in a shallow baking dish. Whisk the orange juice, olive oil, honey, thyme, salt and pepper in a bowl until combined and drizzle over the chicken.

Marinate, covered, in the refrigerator for 8 to 10 hours, turning once. Bake in a preheated 350-degree oven for 30 minutes or until cooked through, basting with the marinade occasionally.

Yield: 4 servings

NUTRIENTS PER SERVING

Calories	258	Cholesterol	78 mg	Fiber	<1 g
Total Fat	10 g	Protein	29 g	Sodium	69 mg
Saturated Fat	2 g	Carbohydrates	12 g	Total Sugar	11 g

DIETARY EXCHANGES: 1 Other Carbohydrate/Sugar, 4 Very Lean Protein, 1 Fat
CARB CHOICES: 1

LET US BE GRATEFUL TO PEOPLE WHO MAKE
US HAPPY; THEY ARE THE CHARMING GARDENERS WHO
MAKE OUR SOULS BLOSSOM.

—MARCEL PROUST

Oven-Crisp Chicken

3 tablespoons all-purpose flour
$1/2$ teaspoon poultry seasoning
$1/4$ teaspoon garlic powder
$1/4$ teaspoon freshly ground pepper
$1 1/2$ cups cornflakes, crushed
1 tablespoon parsley flakes
1 egg white
1 tablespoon water
4 (5-ounce) boneless skinless
    chicken breasts, trimmed

Preheat the oven to 375 degrees. Mix the flour, poultry seasoning, garlic powder and pepper in a sealable plastic bag. Combine the cornflake crumbs and parsley flakes in a shallow dish and mix well. Whisk the egg white and water in a small bowl until blended.

Add the chicken in batches to the flour mixture and seal tightly. Shake until coated. Remove the chicken from the flour mixture, shaking to remove any excess. Dip in the egg wash and coat with the crumb mixture.

Arrange the chicken in a baking pan and lightly spray the chicken with nonstick cooking spray. Bake for 18 to 20 minutes or until the chicken is cooked through.

Yield: 4 servings

NUTRIENTS PER SERVING

Calories	217	Cholesterol	78 mg	Fiber	1 g
Total Fat	3 g	Protein	31 g	Sodium	183 mg
Saturated Fat	1 g	Carbohydrates	14 g	Total Sugar	1 g

DIETARY EXCHANGES: 1 Starch, 4 Very Lean Protein
CARB CHOICES: 1

Raspberry Balsamic Chicken

1 teaspoon canola oil
$1/2$ cup chopped red onion
4 (5-ounce) boneless skinless
 chicken breasts
$1^1/2$ teaspoons minced
 fresh thyme
$1/4$ teaspoon salt

$1/3$ cup sugar-free seedless
 raspberry preserves
2 tablespoons balsamic vinegar
$1/4$ teaspoon salt
$1/4$ teaspoon freshly
 ground pepper

Heat the canola oil in a large nonstick skillet over medium-high heat and add the onion. Sauté for 5 minutes. Sprinkle the chicken with the thyme and $1/4$ teaspoon salt and add to the skillet. Cook for 6 minutes per side or until cooked through. Remove the chicken to a serving platter and cover to keep warm, reserving the pan drippings.

Reduce the heat to medium and stir the preserves, vinegar, $1/4$ teaspoon salt and the pepper into the reserved pan drippings. Cook until the preserves melt, stirring constantly. Spoon the raspberry sauce over the chicken and serve immediately.

Yield: 4 servings

NUTRIENTS PER SERVING

Calories	195	Cholesterol	78 mg	Fiber	<1 g
Total Fat	4 g	Protein	29 g	Sodium	361 mg
Saturated Fat	1 g	Carbohydrates	11 g	Total Sugar	3 g

DIETARY EXCHANGES: 4 Very Lean Protein, 1 Fruit
CARB CHOICES: 1

SUCCESS IS THE ABILITY TO GO FROM FAILURE TO FAILURE
WITHOUT LOSING YOUR ENTHUSIASM.

—WINSTON CHURCHILL

Rosemary Thyme Roasted Turkey

1 (10-pound) turkey
1 tablespoon minced garlic
2 teaspoons freshly ground pepper
1 teaspoon salt
8 sprigs of thyme
3 sprigs of rosemary
3 sprigs of oregano
2 tablespoons olive oil

Preheat the oven to 400 degrees. Remove and discard the giblets from the inside cavity. Rinse the turkey with cold water and pat dry with paper towels. Rub the inside cavity with the garlic and sprinkle with the pepper and salt. Add the sprigs of thyme, rosemary and oregano to the inside cavity and coat the outside surface with the olive oil.

Arrange the turkey in a roasting pan and roast for 15 minutes. Reduce the oven temperature to 325 degrees and roast for 4 hours longer or until a meat thermometer registers 180 degrees. Remove the turkey to a serving platter and let rest for 30 minutes. Remove the skin and slice as desired.

Yield: 16 (5-ounce) servings

NUTRIENTS PER SERVING

Calories	229	Cholesterol	139 mg	Fiber	<1 g
Total Fat	5 g	Protein	42 g	Sodium	240 mg
Saturated Fat	1 g	Carbohydrates	<1 g	Total Sugar	0 g

DIETARY EXCHANGES: 6 Very Lean Meat
CARB CHOICES: 0

Turkey, Squash and Apple Symphony

1 1/2 pounds turkey thighs, skin removed

1 pound acorn squash, cut crosswise into
   1-inch slices

1 pound Rome apples, cut into 1/2-inch slices

1/4 cup apple juice

3 tablespoons brown sugar

1/2 teaspoon ground cinnamon

1/4 teaspoon ground nutmeg

Preheat the oven to 350 degrees. Arrange the turkey on one side of a 9×13-inch baking dish sprayed with nonstick cooking spray. Layer the squash and apples alternately on the other side of the dish. Mix the apple juice, brown sugar, cinnamon and nutmeg in a bowl and pour the apple juice mixture over the turkey and layered squash mixture.

Bake, covered with foil, for 1 hour. Remove the cover and baste with the pan juices. Bake, uncovered, for 15 minutes longer or until a meat thermometer registers 180 degrees.

Yield: 4 servings

NUTRIENTS PER SERVING

Calories	300	Cholesterol	65 mg	Fiber	4 g
Total Fat	9 g	Protein	21 g	Sodium	467 mg
Saturated Fat	3 g	Carbohydrates	35 g	Total Sugar	24 g

DIETARY EXCHANGES: 1 Other Carbohydrate/Sugar, 3 Lean Meat, 1 Fruit
CARB CHOICES: 2

WHEREVER THERE IS A HUMAN BEING, THERE IS
AN OPPORTUNITY FOR KINDNESS.

—SENECA

Turkey Burgers

1 1/2 pounds ground turkey breast
1/4 cup seasoned bread crumbs
1/4 cup (1 ounce) grated Parmesan cheese
1/4 cup minced onion
2 tablespoons skim milk
1 egg white, lightly beaten
2 tablespoons canola oil
6 hamburger buns, heated

Combine the ground turkey, bread crumbs, cheese, onion, skim milk and egg white in a bowl and mix well. Shape the turkey mixture evenly into six patties. Arrange the patties on a baking sheet and freeze for 30 minutes.

Heat the canola oil in a large skillet and add the turkey patties. Cook for approximately 5 minutes per side or until cooked through, turning once. Arrange one turkey patty on each bun and dress with lettuce, tomato and pickles, if desired.

Yield: 6 burgers

NUTRIENTS PER BURGER

Calories	325	Cholesterol	78 mg	Fiber	1 g
Total Fat	8 g	Protein	34 g	Sodium	404 mg
Saturated Fat	2 g	Carbohydrates	26 g	Total Sugar	4 g

DIETARY EXCHANGES: 2 Starch, 4 Very Lean Protein, 1 Fat
CARB CHOICES: 2

Turkey and Black Bean Chili

1 pound ground turkey breast
$1/2$ cup chopped onion
2 (28-ounce) cans no-added-salt diced tomatoes
2 (15-ounce) cans black beans, drained
　and rinsed
1 (4-ounce) can chopped green chiles
1 tablespoon chili powder
1 teaspoon ground cumin
$1/4$ teaspoon garlic powder

Brown the ground turkey with the onion in a stockpot, stirring until the turkey is crumbly; drain. Stir in the undrained tomatoes, beans, green chiles, chili powder, cumin and garlic powder. Bring to a boil, stirring frequently.

Reduce the heat to low and simmer for 30 minutes or until of the desired consistency, stirring occasionally. Ladle into chili bowls.

Yield: 8 servings

NUTRIENTS PER SERVING

Calories	167	Cholesterol	35 mg	Fiber	9 g
Total Fat	1 g	Protein	19 g	Sodium	817 mg
Saturated Fat	<1 g	Carbohydrates	29 g	Total Sugar	9 g

DIETARY EXCHANGES: 1 Starch, 1 Very Lean Meat, 1 Vegetable
CARB CHOICES: 2

CHAMPIONS KEEP PLAYING UNTIL THEY GET IT RIGHT.

—BILLIE JEAN KING

Almost Like Mom's Turkey Loaf

1 pound ground turkey breast
$1/2$ cup quick-cooking oats
$1/2$ cup ketchup
$1/2$ cup chopped mushrooms
$1/4$ cup chopped onion
$1/4$ cup chopped green
   bell pepper
2 eggs, beaten

1 teaspoon Worcestershire sauce
$1/4$ teaspoon sage
$1/4$ teaspoon garlic powder
$1/4$ teaspoon parsley flakes
$1/4$ teaspoon salt
$1/4$ teaspoon freshly
   ground pepper

Preheat the oven to 350 degrees. Combine the ground turkey, oats, ketchup, mushrooms, onion, bell pepper, eggs, Worcestershire sauce, sage, garlic powder, parsley flakes, salt and pepper in a bowl and mix well. Shape the ground turkey mixture into a loaf in a 5×9-inch loaf pan sprayed with nonstick cooking spray.

Bake for 30 to 40 minutes or until a wooden pick inserted in the center comes out clean. Cool slightly and remove to a serving platter. You may freeze and reheat in the microwave, if desired.

Yield: 6 servings

NUTRIENTS PER SERVING

Calories	163	Cholesterol	122 mg	Fiber		1 g
Total Fat	4 g	Protein	20 g	Sodium		383 mg
Saturated Fat	1 g	Carbohydrates	11 g	Total Sugar		5 g

DIETARY EXCHANGES: 1 Starch, 3 Very Lean Protein
CARB CHOICES: 1

> DO NOT GO WHERE THE PATH MAY LEAD, GO INSTEAD
> WHERE THERE IS NO PATH AND LEAVE A TRAIL.
>
> —RALPH WALDO EMERSON

Italian Meat Loaf

1 cup coarsely chopped carrots
1 cup coarsely chopped red onion
$1/4$ cup plain bread crumbs
12 ounces ground turkey breast
1 egg white, lightly beaten
Salt and freshly ground black pepper to taste
1 cup canned crushed tomatoes with liquid
8 black olives, sliced
$1/8$ teaspoon crushed red pepper flakes

Preheat the oven to 450 degrees. Combine the carrots and onion in a microwave-safe bowl and microwave on High for 3 minutes. Mix the carrot mixture, bread crumbs, ground turkey and egg white in a bowl. Season to taste with salt and black pepper.

Shape the turkey mixture into two 3×6-inch loaves on a baking sheet lined with foil and bake for 15 minutes. Combine the tomatoes, olives and red pepper flakes in a microwave-safe bowl and microwave on High for 2 minutes or until heated through and slightly thickened. Arrange one meat loaf on each of two dinner plates and spoon one-half of the tomato mixture over each loaf. Serve immediately.

Yield: 2 (1-loaf) servings

NUTRIENTS PER SERVING

Calories	348	Cholesterol	106 mg	Fiber	6 g
Total Fat	4 g	Protein	45 g	Sodium	516 mg
Saturated Fat	1 g	Carbohydrates	34 g	Total Sugar	.7 g

DIETARY EXCHANGES: 1 Starch, 5 Very Lean Protein, 3 Vegetable
CARB CHOICES: 2

Flounder in Orange Sauce

$1/3$ cup sugar-free orange marmalade
2 tablespoons orange juice
$1/4$ teaspoon ground ginger
$1/3$ cup sliced onion
4 (4-ounce) flounder fillets

Preheat the oven to 400 degrees. Mix the marmalade, orange juice and ginger in a saucepan and cook over medium heat until heated through, stirring occasionally. Remove from the heat and stir in the onion.

Arrange the fillets in a single layer in a 9×13-inch baking pan sprayed with nonstick cooking spray. Spoon the marmalade mixture over the fillets and bake for 10 minutes or until the fillets flake easily.

Yield: 4 servings

NUTRIENTS PER SERVING

Calories	112	Cholesterol	53 mg	Fiber	<1 g
Total Fat	1 g	Protein	19 g	Sodium	83 mg
Saturated Fat	<1 g	Carbohydrates	8 g	Total Sugar	1 g

DIETARY EXCHANGES: 3 Very Lean Protein, $1/2$ Fruit
CARB CHOICES: $1/2$

DON'T START LIVING TOMORROW; TOMORROW
NEVER ARRIVES. START WORKING ON YOUR DREAMS
AND AMBITIONS TODAY.

Grouper with Peppers

1 tablespoon olive oil
1 onion, sliced
1 green bell pepper, cut into strips
1 red bell pepper, cut into strips
2 tomatoes, chopped
6 garlic cloves, minced
6 (6-ounce) grouper fillets
1 teaspoon salt
$1/4$ teaspoon freshly ground pepper
4 ounces feta cheese, crumbled
2 tablespoons chopped fresh parsley

Preheat the oven to 375 degrees. Heat the olive oil in a skillet over medium heat and add the onion, bell peppers, tomatoes and garlic. Sauté until the onion is tender and remove from the heat. Arrange the fillets in a single layer in a baking dish and sprinkle with the salt and pepper. Spoon the sautéed vegetables over the fillets.

Bake for 20 minutes or until the fillets flake easily. Sprinkle with the cheese and parsley and bake for 5 minutes longer. Serve immediately.

Yield: 6 servings

NUTRIENTS PER SERVING

Calories	261	Cholesterol	81 mg	Fiber	2 g
Total Fat	8 g	Protein	38 g	Sodium	675 mg
Saturated Fat	4 g	Carbohydrates	8 g	Total Sugar	4 g

DIETARY EXCHANGES: 5 Very Lean Protein, 1 Vegetable, 1 Fat
CARB CHOICES: $1/2$

Salsa-Topped Tilapia

PHOTOGRAPH FOR THIS RECIPE APPEARS ON PAGE 49.

4 (4-ounce) tilapia or orange roughy fillets, $1/2$ inch thick	$1/4$ cup chopped onion
1 cup chopped tomato	$1/4$ teaspoon salt
$1/2$ cup chopped green bell pepper	$1/4$ cup canned chicken broth or dry white wine
2 tablespoons chopped fresh parsley	Lemon wedges for garnish
	Sprigs of flat-leaf parsley for garnish

Heat a skillet sprayed with nonstick cooking spray over medium heat. Arrange the fillets in the hot skillet and cook for 4 to 6 minutes or until the fillets flake easily, turning once. Remove to a heated platter, reserving the pan drippings.

Mix the tomato, bell pepper, parsley, onion and salt with the reserved pan drippings. Cook for 3 to 5 minutes or until the bell pepper and onion are tender-crisp, stirring constantly. Add the broth and cook until heated through, stirring constantly. Spoon the salsa mixture over the fillets and garnish with lemon wedges and parsley. Serve immediately.

Yield: 4 servings

NUTRIENTS PER SERVING

Calories	135	Cholesterol	80 mg	Fiber	1 g
Total Fat	3 g	Protein	24 g	Sodium	206 mg
Saturated Fat	1 g	Carbohydrates	4 g	Total Sugar	2 g

DIETARY EXCHANGES: 2 Lean Meat, 1 Vegetable
CARB CHOICES: 0

BECOME ADDICTED TO CONSTANT AND
NEVER-ENDING SELF-IMPROVEMENT.

—ANTHONY J. D'ANGELO

Baked Honey Dijon Salmon

$1/2$ cup lemon juice
$1/2$ cup white wine or apple juice
2 pounds salmon fillets, cut into 8 equal portions
$1/4$ cup ($1/2$ stick) butter, melted
3 tablespoons Dijon mustard
$1 1/2$ tablespoons honey
Salt and freshly ground pepper to taste
$1/4$ cup dry bread crumbs
$1/4$ cup finely chopped almonds
2 tablespoons chopped fresh parsley

Whisk the lemon juice and wine in a small bowl. Arrange the salmon in a single layer in a 9×13-inch baking dish and drizzle with the lemon juice mixture. Marinate, covered, in the refrigerator for 3 to 4 hours, turning occasionally.

Preheat the oven to 375 degrees. Mix the butter, Dijon mustard, honey, salt and pepper in a bowl until blended. Combine the bread crumbs, almonds and parsley in a bowl and mix well. Brush the salmon with the butter mixture and sprinkle the tops with the bread crumb mixture. Bake for 12 to 15 minutes or until the salmon flakes easily.

Yield: 8 servings

NUTRIENTS PER SERVING

Calories	326	Cholesterol	97 mg	Fiber	1 g
Total Fat	19 g	Protein	28 g	Sodium	271 mg
Saturated Fat	6 g	Carbohydrates	9 g	Total Sugar	4 g

DIETARY EXCHANGES: 1 Other Carbohydrate/Sugar, 4 Very Lean Protein, 2 Fat
CARB CHOICES: 1

Sole and Spinach Pie

1 (10-ounce) package frozen
  chopped spinach,
  thawed and drained
16 ounces fresh or thawed
  frozen sole, or any other
  white fish fillets
Salt to taste
2 eggs, lightly beaten

1 tablespoon chopped fresh
  chives or minced onion
2 tablespoons grated
  Parmesan cheese
Ground nutmeg to taste
Freshly ground pepper to taste
1 tablespoon butter

Press the excess moisture from the spinach. Simmer the fillets in enough salted water to cover in a saucepan for 10 minutes or until the fillets flake easily; drain.

Preheat the oven to 400 degrees. Flake the fillets into a 9-inch pie plate sprayed with nonstick cooking spray. Combine the spinach, eggs, chives, cheese, nutmeg, pepper and salt in a bowl and mix well. Pour over the fish and dot with the butter. Bake for 20 minutes. Serve hot or chilled.

Yield: 6 servings

NUTRIENTS PER SERVING

Calories	124	Cholesterol	112 mg	Fiber	1 g
Total Fat	5 g	Protein	17 g	Sodium	152 mg
Saturated Fat	2 g	Carbohydrates	2 g	Total Sugar	1 g

DIETARY EXCHANGES: 2 Very Lean Protein, 1 Fat
CARB CHOICES: 0

BIG SHOTS ARE ONLY LITTLE SHOTS WHO KEEP SHOOTING.

—CHRISTOPHER MORLEY

Spicy Shrimp Pasta

8 ounces whole wheat penne pasta
$1/4$ cup olive oil
1 pound medium shrimp, peeled and deveined
1 green bell pepper, cut into strips
1 yellow bell pepper, cut into strips
1 cup sliced fresh mushrooms
3 garlic cloves, minced
1 tablespoon dried basil, crushed
2 tomatoes, chopped
$3/4$ cup picante sauce
$1/4$ cup (1 ounce) grated Parmesan cheese

Cook the pasta using the package directions and drain. Cover to keep warm. Heat the olive oil in a large nonstick skillet over medium-high heat and add the shrimp, bell peppers, mushrooms, garlic and basil.

Cook for 3 to 4 minutes or until the shrimp turn pink, stirring frequently. Stir in the tomatoes and picante sauce and simmer for 2 to 3 minutes, stirring occasionally. Add the pasta and toss to mix. Spoon the shrimp mixture into a serving bowl and sprinkle with the cheese.

Yield: 4 servings

NUTRIENTS PER SERVING

Calories	477	Cholesterol	172 mg	Fiber	8 g
Total Fat	17 g	Protein	29 g	Sodium	626 mg
Saturated Fat	3 g	Carbohydrates	53 g	Total Sugar	6 g

DIETARY EXCHANGES: 3 Starch, 3 Very Lean Protein, 1 Vegetable, 2 Fat
CARB CHOICES: 3

Pasta with Red Pepper Sauce

PHOTOGRAPH FOR THIS RECIPE APPEARS ON PAGE 52.

4 red bell peppers, chopped
2 carrots, finely chopped
1 tablespoon olive oil
2 cups canned undrained
    Italian-seasoned tomatoes
1 tablespoon chopped fresh basil, or
    1 teaspoon dried basil
$1/2$ pear, chopped
Minced garlic to taste
Salt and freshly ground pepper to taste
8 ounces whole wheat penne pasta,
    cooked and drained
$1/4$ cup (1 ounce) grated Parmesan cheese
Fresh basil leaves for garnish

Sauté the bell peppers and carrots in the olive oil in a nonstick skillet for 4 to 5 minutes or until tender. Stir in the tomatoes, chopped basil, pear, garlic, salt and pepper. Simmer for 45 minutes, stirring occasionally. Toss the tomato sauce with the pasta in a bowl and sprinkle with the cheese. Garnish with fresh basil leaves and serve immediately.

Yield: 4 servings

NUTRIENTS PER SERVING

Calories	345	Cholesterol	4 mg	Fiber	10 g
Total Fat	7 g	Protein	12 g	Sodium	300 mg
Saturated Fat	1 g	Carbohydrates	60 g	Total Sugar	13 g

DIETARY EXCHANGES: 4 Starch, 1 Fat
CARB CHOICES: 4

Southwestern Tomato Pasta

3 or 4 small ripe tomatoes
2 tablespoons extra-virgin olive oil
3 garlic cloves, minced
3 tablespoons chopped fresh cilantro
1 tablespoon fresh lime juice
$1/2$ teaspoon chili powder
$1/4$ teaspoon salt
$1/4$ teaspoon white pepper
8 ounces whole wheat angel hair pasta
2 ounces feta cheese, crumbled

Peel and coarsely chop the tomatoes over a bowl to catch the juice. Stir in the olive oil, garlic, cilantro, lime juice, chili powder, salt and white pepper. Let stand, covered, at room temperature for 1 hour.

Cook the pasta using the package directions and drain. Spoon the warm pasta onto a serving platter and top with the tomato mixture. Sprinkle with the cheese.

Yield: 4 servings

NUTRIENTS PER SERVING

Calories	335	Cholesterol	13 mg	Fiber	6 g
Total Fat	12 g	Protein	10 g	Sodium	326 mg
Saturated Fat	3 g	Carbohydrates	48 g	Total Sugar	5 g

DIETARY EXCHANGES: 3 Starch, 2 Fat
CARB CHOICES: 3

ONE WORD FREES US OF ALL THE WEIGHT AND
PAIN OF LIFE; THAT WORD IS LOVE.

—SOPHOCLES

Desserts Contents

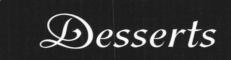
Desserts

Old-Fashioned
Bread Pudding
page 104

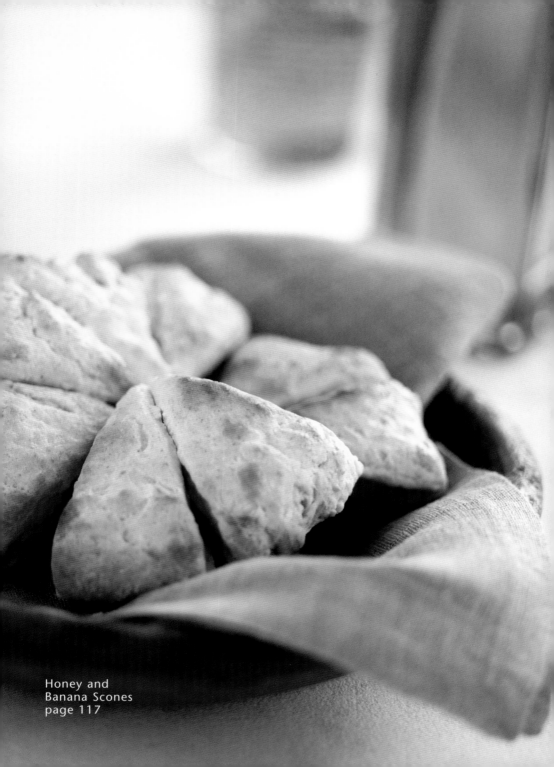

Honey and
Banana Scones
page 117

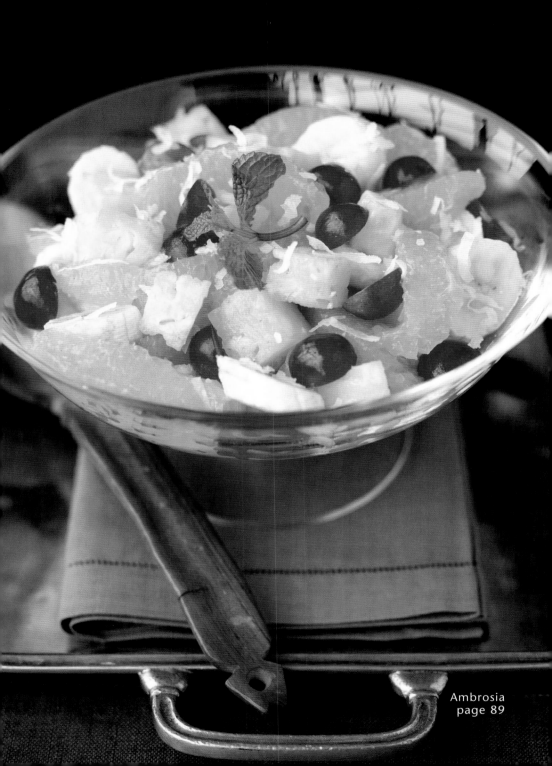

Ambrosia
page 89

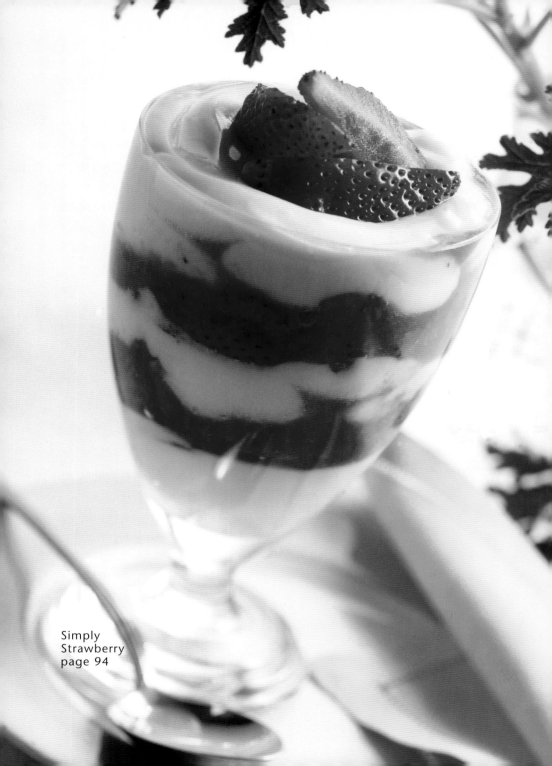

Simply
Strawberry
page 94

Ambrosia

PHOTOGRAPH FOR THIS RECIPE APPEARS ON PAGE 87.

1 (20-ounce) can juice-pack
   pineapple chunks, drained
1 (11-ounce) can mandarin oranges, drained
1 banana, sliced
1 cup miniature marshmallows
$1^{1}/_{2}$ cups seedless red grapes
$^{1}/_{2}$ cup flaked coconut
$^{1}/_{2}$ cup chopped pecans
1 cup vanilla nonfat yogurt
1 sprig of mint for garnish

Gently mix the pineapple, mandarin oranges, banana, marshmallows, grapes, coconut and pecans in a serving bowl. Fold in the yogurt and chill, covered, until serving time. Garnish with a sprig of mint.

Yield: 8 servings

NUTRIENTS PER SERVING

Calories	221	Cholesterol	<1 mg	Fiber	3 g
Total Fat	7 g	Protein	3 g	Sodium	42 mg
Saturated Fat	2 g	Carbohydrates	40 g	Total Sugar	34 g

DIETARY EXCHANGES: 1 Other Carbohydrate/Sugar, 1 Fruit, 1 Fat
CARB CHOICES: 2

OUR HEALTH ALWAYS SEEMS MUCH MORE
VALUABLE AFTER WE LOSE IT.

Honey Crunch Baked Apples

6 large baking apples, cored and peeled
$1/3$ cup low-fat granola
$1/3$ cup chopped dates
$1/4$ cup chopped walnuts
2 teaspoons lemon juice
$1/2$ teaspoon ground cinnamon
$1/4$ teaspoon ground nutmeg
$1/3$ cup honey
$3/4$ cup unsweetened apple juice
3 tablespoons butter, melted

Preheat the oven to 350 degrees. Arrange the apples in a 9-inch baking pan. Mix the granola, dates, walnuts, lemon juice, cinnamon and nutmeg in a bowl and stir in 3 tablespoons of the honey. Pack the granola mixture lightly into the centers of the apples.

Mix the remaining honey, the apple juice and butter in a bowl and drizzle over the apples. Bake, covered, for 30 minutes. Remove the cover and bake for 35 minutes longer, basting with the pan juices occasionally. Serve warm or at room temprature.

Yield: 6 apples

NUTRIENTS PER APPLE

Calories	279	Cholesterol	15 mg	Fiber	3 g
Total Fat	10 g	Protein	2 g	Sodium	52 mg
Saturated Fat	4 g	Carbohydrates	52 g	Total Sugar	43 g

DIETARY EXCHANGES: 1 Starch, 1 Other Carbohydrate/Sugar, 1 Fruit, 2 Fat
CARB CHOICES: 3

Banana Pops

2 bananas, cut crosswise into halves
$1/4$ cup crisp rice cereal
1 tablespoon toasted shredded coconut
1 tablespoon finely chopped peanuts
$1/4$ teaspoon ground nutmeg
2 teaspoons light corn syrup

Insert a wooden popsicle stick in the cut end of each banana half and arrange on a baking sheet. Freeze for 1 hour or until firm.

Combine the cereal, coconut, peanuts and nutmeg in a shallow dish and mix well. Brush the bananas with the syrup and coat with the cereal mixture. Wrap the coated bananas individually in plastic wrap and freeze for 2 hours or longer.

Yield: 4 pops

NUTRIENTS PER POP

Calories	88	Cholesterol	0 mg	Fiber	2 g
Total Fat	2 g	Protein	1 g	Sodium	19 mg
Saturated Fat	1 g	Carbohydrates	18 g	Total Sugar	9 g

DIETARY EXCHANGES: 1 Other Carbohydrate/Sugar
CARB CHOICES: 1

> SMILE AT EACH OTHER, SMILE AT YOUR WIFE,
> SMILE AT YOUR HUSBAND, SMILE AT YOUR CHILDREN,
> SMILE AT EACH OTHER—IT DOESN'T MATTER
> WHO IT IS—AND THAT WILL HELP YOU TO GROW UP IN
> GREATER LOVE FOR EACH OTHER.
>
> —MOTHER TERESA

Cranberry Coconut Delight

1 (20-ounce) can juice-pack crushed pineapple
1 large package sugar-free cran-raspberry gelatin
1 cup shredded coconut
2 cups buttermilk
1 cup pecan pieces
12 ounces nonfat whipped topping

Bring the undrained pineapple to a boil in a large saucepan over medium-high heat. Remove from the heat and add the gelatin, stirring until dissolved. Let stand until cool.

Stir the coconut, buttermilk and pecans into the gelatin mixture. Fold in the whipped topping. Spoon into a 9×13-inch dish and chill, covered, until set.

Yield: 15 servings

NUTRIENTS PER SERVING

Calories	170	Cholesterol	1 mg	Fiber	2 g
Total Fat	8 g	Protein	4 g	Sodium	146 mg
Saturated Fat	2 g	Carbohydrates	26 g	Total Sugar	10 g

DIETARY EXCHANGES: 1 Starch, 1 Fruit, 1 Fat
CARB CHOICES: 2

DO NOT FEAR THE WINDS OF ADVERSITY. REMEMBER: A KITE RISES AGAINST THE WIND RATHER THAN WITH IT.

Lemon Berry Whip

1 small package sugar-free lemon gelatin
1 cup boiling water
5 ice cubes
1 2/3 cups nonfat whipped topping
1 cup chopped fresh strawberries

Whisk the gelatin into the boiling water in a heatproof bowl until dissolved. Add the ice cubes and stir until melted. Chill, covered, in the refrigerator until partially set.

Beat the gelatin in a mixing bowl until doubled in bulk. Fold in three-fourths of the whipped topping and then fold in the strawberries. Spoon the strawberry mixture evenly into dessert goblets and chill, covered, in the refrigerator. Top evenly with the remaining whipped topping just before serving.

Yield: 8 (1-cup) servings

NUTRIENTS PER SERVING

Calories	37	Cholesterol	0 mg	Fiber	<1 g
Total Fat	<1 g	Protein	1 g	Sodium	38 mg
Saturated Fat	0 g	Carbohydrates	7 g	Total Sugar	3 g

DIETARY EXCHANGES: 1 Vegetable
CARB CHOICES: 1/2

Simply Strawberry

PHOTOGRAPH FOR THIS RECIPE APPEARS ON PAGE 88.

1 tablespoon sugar
1 teaspoon balsamic vinegar
1 quart fresh strawberries, sliced
5 cups frozen no-sugar-added vanilla ice cream

Combine the sugar and vinegar in a bowl and mix well. Drizzle over the strawberries in a bowl and toss to coat. Chill, covered, for 30 minutes. Reserve some of the strawberry mixture for the topping.

Layer the ice cream and remaining strawberry mixture equally in ten stemmed dessert goblets, beginning and ending with the ice cream. Top with the reserved strawberry mixture and serve immediately.

For a smoother sauce, process one-half of the strawberry mixture in a blender or food processor until puréed and mix with the remaining sliced strawberry mixture. Proceed as directed above.

Yield: 10 servings

NUTRIENTS PER SERVING

Calories	114	Cholesterol	0 mg	Fiber	1 g
Total Fat	<1 g	Protein	3 g	Sodium	51 mg
Saturated Fat	<1 g	Carbohydrates	25 g	Total Sugar	8 g

DIETARY EXCHANGES: 1 Fruit, 1 Milk
CARB CHOICES: 2

NEVER BE AFRAID TO TRY SOMETHING NEW.
REMEMBER, AMATEURS BUILT THE ARK. PROFESSIONALS
BUILT THE TITANIC.

Peach Meringue with Raspberries

4 fresh peaches, peeled and cut into halves
3 egg whites
1 tablespoon honey, heated
2 (10-ounce) packages frozen
    unsweetened raspberries, thawed

Preheat the oven to 450 degrees. Arrange the peaches cut side up in a shallow baking dish sprayed with nonstick cooking spray. Beat the egg whites in a mixing bowl until soft peaks form. Add the honey gradually, beating constantly until stiff peaks form.

Mound the meringue evenly in the centers of the peach halves and bake for 4 to 5 minutes or until light brown. Spread the raspberries in a shallow dish and arrange the peach halves over the raspberries. You may substitute one drained 29-ounce can juice-pack peaches for the fresh peaches.

Yield: 8 servings

NUTRIENTS PER SERVING

Calories	106	Cholesterol	0 mg	Fiber	4 g
Total Fat	<1 g	Protein	2 g	Sodium	22 mg
Saturated Fat	<1 g	Carbohydrates	25 g	Total Sugar	9 g

DIETARY EXCHANGES: 2 Fruit
CARB CHOICES: 2

Vanilla-Poached Pears

3 firm pears
2 lemon wedges
4 cups water
3 tablespoons vanilla extract
2 tablespoons honey
3 tablespoons nonfat whipped topping

Peel and core the pears, leaving the stems intact. Cut a thin slice from the bottom of each pear so the pears will stand upright. Rub the surface of the pears with the lemon wedges to prevent browning.

Bring the water, vanilla and honey to a boil in a large saucepan over high heat. Reduce the heat and add the pears upright. Cook, covered, for 15 to 20 minutes or until tender. Remove the pears from the cooking liquid and cool slightly. Arrange one pear on each of three dessert plates and top each with 1 tablespoon of the whipped topping.

Yield: 3 pears

NUTRIENTS PER PEAR

Calories	189	Cholesterol	0 mg	Fiber	4 g
Total Fat	1 g	Protein	1 g	Sodium	4 mg
Saturated Fat	0 g	Carbohydrates	40 g	Total Sugar	31 g

DIETARY EXCHANGES: 1 Other Carbohydrate/Sugar, 1 Fruit
CARB CHOICES: 2

Coffee and Cream Delight

1 envelope unflavored gelatin
$1/2$ cup cold coffee
2 cups boiling strong coffee
$1/2$ cup Splenda
6 tablespoons nonfat whipped topping

Soften the gelatin in the cold coffee in a heatproof bowl. Stir in the boiling coffee and artificial sweetener. Cool slightly and pour into dessert goblets. Chill until set. Top each serving with 1 tablespoon of the whipped topping.

Yield: 6 servings

NUTRIENTS PER SERVING

Calories	21	Cholesterol	0 mg	Fiber	0 g
Total Fat	<1 g	Protein	1 g	Sodium	7 mg
Saturated Fat	0 g	Carbohydrates	4 g	Total Sugar	1 g

DIETARY EXCHANGES: Free
CARB CHOICES: 0

> THE EARLY BIRD MAY GET THE WORM, BUT THE
> SECOND MOUSE GETS THE CHEESE.
>
> —STEVEN WRIGHT

Instant Boiled Custard

2 small packages sugar-free vanilla
  instant pudding mix
8 cups skim milk
1 teaspoon vanilla extract
1 (15-ounce) can fat-free sweetened
  condensed milk

Combine the pudding mix and skim milk in a mixing bowl and beat until blended. Add the vanilla and condensed milk and beat until smooth. Chill, covered, in the refrigerator. Ladle into punch cups or mugs.

Yield: 10 (1-cup) servings

NUTRIENTS PER SERVING

Calories	203	Cholesterol	7 mg	Fiber	0 g
Total Fat	<1 g	Protein	10 g	Sodium	361 mg
Saturated Fat	<1 g	Carbohydrates	40 g	Total Sugar	36 g

DIETARY EXCHANGES: 2 Other Carbohydrate/Sugar, 1 Milk
CARB CHOICES: 3

LOVE IS LIKE PLAYING THE PIANO. FIRST YOU
MUST LEARN TO PLAY BY THE RULES; THEN YOU MUST
FORGET THE RULES AND PLAY FROM YOUR HEART.

Baked Pumpkin Custard

$1/2$ cup graham cracker crumbs

1 (15-ounce) can pumpkin purée

1 (12-ounce) can evaporated skim milk

$1/4$ cup packed brown sugar

2 egg whites

1 egg

1 teaspoon ground cinnamon

$1/4$ teaspoon ground allspice

1 teaspoon vanilla extract

9 tablespoons nonfat whipped topping

Preheat the oven to 325 degrees. Sprinkle the graham cracker crumbs over the bottom of an 8×8-inch baking pan sprayed with nonstick cooking spray. Beat the pumpkin, evaporated skim milk, brown sugar, egg whites, egg, cinnamon, allspice and vanilla in a mixing bowl until blended.

Spread the pumpkin mixture in the prepared pan and bake for 50 to 60 minutes or until a knife inserted in the center comes out clean. Cool in the pan on a wire rack for 20 minutes. Spoon the custard evenly into individual dessert bowls and top each with 1 tablespoon whipped topping.

Yield: 9 servings

NUTRIENTS PER SERVING

Calories	108	Cholesterol	25 mg	Fiber	2 g
Total Fat	1 g	Protein	5 g	Sodium	99 mg
Saturated Fat	<1 g	Carbohydrates	19 g	Total Sugar	14 g

DIETARY EXCHANGES: 1 Milk
CARB CHOICES: 1

Chocolate Mousse Surprise

$1^1/_2$ cups crushed cornflakes
3 tablespoons honey
8 ounces light cream
   cheese, softened
1 cup confectioners' sugar
16 ounces lite whipped topping
3 cups skim milk

2 large packages sugar-free
   fat-free chocolate fudge
   instant pudding mix
$1/_2$ cup fat-free fudge topping
$1/_4$ cup semisweet
   chocolate chips

Preheat the oven to 350 degrees. Toss the cornflake crumbs and honey in a bowl and press over the bottom of a 9×13-inch baking dish sprayed with nonstick cooking spray. Bake for 10 minutes. Let stand until cool.

Beat the cream cheese and confectioners' sugar in a mixing bowl until smooth. Fold in half the whipped topping. Beat the skim milk and pudding mix in a mixing bowl until thickened and fold into the cream cheese mixture. Spread the cream cheese mixture over the baked layer and top with dollops of the fudge topping. Spread with the remaining whipped topping and sprinkle with the chocolate chips. Chill, covered, until serving time.

Yield: 12 servings

NUTRIENTS PER SERVING

Calories	292	Cholesterol	8 mg	Fiber	<1 g
Total Fat	7 g	Protein	6 g	Sodium	271 mg
Saturated Fat	6 g	Carbohydrates	53 g	Total Sugar	23 g

DIETARY EXCHANGES: 2 Other Carbohydrate/Sugar, 1 Milk
CARB CHOICES: 3

BY PERSEVERANCE THE SNAIL REACHED THE ARK.

—CHARLES HADDON SPURGEON

Two-Berry Mousse

2 cups frozen unsweetened
   loose-pack raspberries, thawed
1 1/2 cups frozen unsweetened
   loose-pack strawberries,
   thawed
1 large package sugar-free
   raspberry gelatin

1 cup boiling water
1/2 cup light sour cream
2 tablespoons lemon juice
1 pint strawberry or vanilla
   frozen yogurt
1/2 cup nonfat whipped topping

Combine the raspberries and strawberries in a blender and process until puréed. Strain, discarding the seeds. Dissolve the gelatin in the boiling water in a heatproof bowl and cool slightly.

Combine the gelatin, sour cream, lemon juice and yogurt in a blender and process until smooth. Fold the gelatin mixture into the puréed berries in a bowl. Spoon the mousse into eight dessert goblets or dessert bowls and chill for 4 to 6 hours or until set. Top each with 1 tablespoon of the whipped topping before serving.

Yield: 8 servings

NUTRIENTS PER SERVING

Calories	195	Cholesterol	30 mg	Fiber	3 g
Total Fat	3 g	Protein	5 g	Sodium	100 mg
Saturated Fat	2 g	Carbohydrates	36 g	Total Sugar	5 g

DIETARY EXCHANGES: 1 Other Carbohydrate/Sugar, 1 Fruit, 1 Fat
CARB CHOICES: 2

Lemon Strawberry Parfaits

1 envelope unflavored gelatin
$1/2$ cup cold water
$3/4$ cup Splenda
$1/2$ cup fresh lemon juice
1 egg

1 tablespoon extra-light olive oil
2 teaspoons grated lemon zest
$1 1/3$ cups plain fat-free yogurt
2 cups sliced fresh strawberries

Sprinkle the gelatin over $1/4$ cup of the cold water in a small bowl. Let stand for 5 minutes and stir. Whisk the remaining $1/4$ cup cold water, artificial sweetener, lemon juice, egg, olive oil and lemon zest in a saucepan until combined.

Cook over low heat for 5 minutes or until the mixture is hot, stirring constantly. Mix in the gelatin mixture and cook for 1 minute longer or until the gelatin dissolves. Pour the lemon mixture into a heatproof bowl and let stand until room temperature, stirring occasionally. Whisk in the yogurt.

Reserve the desired amount of strawberry slices for the top of each parfait. Layer the lemon mousse and remaining strawberries alternately in eight stemmed goblets or parfait glasses, beginning and ending with the lemon mousse. Top each parfait with equal amounts of the reserved strawberry slices. Chill, covered, in the refrigerator until set.

Yield: 8 servings

NUTRIENTS PER SERVING

Calories	70	Cholesterol	27 mg	Fiber	1 g
Total Fat	2 g	Protein	4 g	Sodium	34 mg
Saturated Fat	<1 g	Carbohydrates	10 g	Total Sugar	5 g

DIETARY EXCHANGES: 1 Fruit
CARB CHOICES: 1

Strawberry Ricotta Dream Dessert

1 envelope unflavored gelatin
$3/4$ cup skim milk
1 cup low-fat ricotta cheese
1 cup 1% cottage cheese
$1/2$ cup Splenda or granulated
  artificial sweetener

1 teaspoon vanilla extract
$1/2$ cup frozen unsweetened
  strawberries, thawed
$1/4$ cup miniature semisweet
  chocolate chips

Sprinkle the gelatin over $1/4$ cup of the skim milk in a blender and let stand for 2 minutes. Bring the remaining $1/2$ cup skim milk to a boil in a saucepan and add to the blender. Process at low speed for 2 minutes or until the gelatin dissolves. Add the ricotta cheese, cottage cheese, artificial sweetener and vanilla to the gelatin mixture and process at high speed for 2 minutes or until blended. Pour equal amounts of the mixture into two separate bowls.

Process the strawberries in a blender until puréed; strain, if desired. Stir the strawberry purée into one bowl of the pudding. Chill both bowls of pudding for 3 hours or until set and whisk until smooth. Stir the chocolate chips into the plain pudding. Spoon the pudding mixtures side-by-side into six dessert goblets and serve immediately.

Yield: 6 servings

NUTRIENTS PER SERVING

Calories	147	Cholesterol	15 mg	Fiber	<1 g
Total Fat	5 g	Protein	12 g	Sodium	269 mg
Saturated Fat	3 g	Carbohydrates	14 g	Total Sugar	4 g

DIETARY EXCHANGES: 1 Milk, 1 Fat
CARB CHOICES: 1

CHARACTER CONSISTS OF WHAT YOU DO ON
THE THIRD AND FOURTH TRIES.

—JOHN ALBERT MICHENER

Old-Fashioned Bread Pudding

PHOTOGRAPH FOR THIS RECIPE APPEARS ON PAGE 85.

1 cup dry bread crumbs
$1^1/2$ cups skim milk
$1/2$ cup raisins
2 eggs, lightly beaten
1 teaspoon vanilla extract

$1/2$ teaspoon ground cinnamon
8 envelopes artificial sweetener
Nonfat whipped topping
  for garnish

Preheat the oven to 325 degrees. Soak the bread crumbs in the skim milk in a large bowl for 5 minutes. Add the raisins, eggs, vanilla, cinnamon and artificial sweetener to the milk mixture one at a time, mixing well after each addition.

Pour the pudding mixture into a 9×9-inch baking dish and bake for 50 minutes or until brown and set. Garnish each serving with a dollop of whipped topping.

Yield: 4 servings

NUTRIENTS PER SERVING

Calories	236	Cholesterol	108 mg	Fiber	2 g
Total Fat	4 g	Protein	10 g	Sodium	273 mg
Saturated Fat	1 g	Carbohydrates	40 g	Total Sugar	19 g

DIETARY EXCHANGES: 1 Starch, 1 Medium Fat Meat, 1 Fruit
CARB CHOICES: 3

Tiramisù

PHOTOGRAPH FOR THIS RECIPE APPEARS ON PAGE 4.

$2/3$ cup strong coffee
$1/3$ cup maple syrup
16 ladyfingers, split
3 ounces fat-free cream
   cheese, softened

$1/2$ cup fat-free sour cream
$1/2$ cup maple syrup
12 ounces nonfat
   whipped topping
1 teaspoon baking cocoa

Mix the coffee and $1/3$ cup maple syrup in a bowl and drizzle over the ladyfingers. Line the bottom of an 8×8-inch dish with one-half of the ladyfingers. Beat the cream cheese, sour cream and $1/2$ cup maple syrup in a bowl until smooth. Fold in the whipped topping.

Spread half the cream cheese mixture over the ladyfingers. Top with the remaining ladyfingers and cream cheese mixture. Chill, covered, until serving time. Sift the baking cocoa over the top just before serving.

Yield: 9 servings

NUTRIENTS PER SERVING

Calories	234	Cholesterol	70 mg	Fiber	<1 g
Total Fat	2 g	Protein	4 g	Sodium	108 mg
Saturated Fat	1 g	Carbohydrates	48 g	Total Sugar	23 g

DIETARY EXCHANGES: 1 Starch, 2 Other Carbohydrate/Sugar
CARB CHOICES: 3

> ANY ACTIVITY BECOMES CREATIVE WHEN THE DOER CARES
> ABOUT DOING IT RIGHT, OR BETTER.
>
> —JOHN UPDIKE

Peachy Swiss Cheese Strata

4 slices whole wheat bread,
cut into 1/4-inch cubes
8 dried peaches, chopped
6 ounces Swiss cheese,
cut into 1/4-inch cubes
1 cup liquid egg substitute

1 (12-ounce) can evaporated
skim milk
1 cup peach fat-free yogurt
2 tablespoons Splenda
2 teaspoons ground cinnamon
2 teaspoons vanilla extract

Layer the bread cubes, dried peaches and cheese one-half at a time in a buttered 7×11-inch baking dish. Combine the egg substitute, evaporated skim milk, yogurt, artificial sweetener, cinnamon and vanilla in a bowl and mix well.

Pour the yogurt mixture over the prepared layers and chill, covered, for 8 to 10 hours. Bring to room temperature and place the baking dish on the middle oven rack in a cold oven. Turn the oven temperature to 300 degrees and bake for 1 hour or until light brown and the liquid is absorbed.

Yield: 6 servings

NUTRIENTS PER SERVING

Calories	304	Cholesterol	30 mg	Fiber	3 g
Total Fat	10 g	Protein	21 g	Sodium	331 mg
Saturated Fat	6 g	Carbohydrates	32 g	Total Sugar	19 g

DIETARY EXCHANGES: 2 Medium Fat Meat, 1 Fruit, 1 Milk
CARB CHOICES: 2

SOMETIMES THE HEART SEES WHAT IS INVISIBLE TO THE EYE.

—H. JACKSON BROWN, JR.

Blueberry Cheesecake

PHOTOGRAPH FOR THIS RECIPE APPEARS ON THE COVER.

1 cup crushed
   reduced-fat Triscuits
$1/4$ cup ($1/2$ stick) butter or
   margarine, softened
$1^1/2$ teaspoons Splenda or
   granulated artificial sweetener
16 ounces light cream
   cheese, softened
1 teaspoon vanilla extract

1 tablespoon Splenda or
   granulated artificial sweetener
3 eggs
2 cups fat-free sour cream
2 teaspoons Splenda or
   granulated artificial sweetener
1 teaspoon vanilla extract
$1^1/2$ cups fresh blueberries

Combine the cracker crumbs, butter and $1^1/2$ teaspoons artificial sweetener in a bowl and mix well. Press the crumb mixture over the bottom and up the side of a 9-inch pie plate sprayed with nonstick cooking spray.

Preheat the oven to 375 degrees. Beat the cream cheese in a mixing bowl at medium speed for 2 to 3 minutes, scraping the bowl occasionally. Add 1 teaspoon vanilla and 1 tablespoon artificial sweetener gradually, beating constantly until blended. Beat in the eggs one at a time.

Spread the cream cheese mixture in the prepared pie plate and bake for 20 minutes. Remove from the oven and cool for 15 minutes. Increase the oven temperature to 475 degrees. Mix the sour cream, 2 teaspoons artificial sweetener and 1 teaspoon vanilla in a bowl and spread over the baked layer, sealing to the edge. Bake for 10 minutes longer. Let stand until cool and chill, covered, until serving time. Top with the blueberries just before serving.

Yield: 8 servings

NUTRIENTS PER SERVING

Calories	266	Cholesterol	114 mg	Fiber	1 g
Total Fat	13 g	Protein	13 g	Sodium	360 mg
Saturated Fat	7 g	Carbohydrates	22 g	Total Sugar	8 g

DIETARY EXCHANGES: 1 Medium Fat Meat, 1 Milk, 2 Fat
CARB CHOICES: 1

Chocolate Wafer Cheesecake

Chocolate Wafer Crust
1 (9-ounce) package dark
chocolate wafers
1 egg white, lightly beaten

Filling
2 cups nonfat cottage cheese
16 ounces light cream cheese,
cut into chunks

6 egg whites
$1/4$ cup all-purpose flour
2 teaspoons vanilla extract
$3/4$ cup (or less) Splenda or
granulated artificial sweetener
14 dark chocolate wafers,
broken into halves

For the crust, preheat the oven to 300 degrees. Process the wafers in a blender until ground. Add 1 egg white and process until moistened. Press the crumb mixture over the bottom and $1/2$ inch up the side of a 9-inch springform pan. Bake for 20 minutes. Let stand until cool. Maintain the oven temperature.

For the filling, combine the cottage cheese, cream cheese, egg whites, flour, vanilla and artificial sweetener in a blender and process until smooth. Spread two-thirds of the cheese mixture over the cooled baked layer and arrange the wafer halves over the top, overlapping to cover. Spread with the remaining cheese mixture, sealing to the edge of the pan.

Place the pan on a baking sheet and bake for 25 to 30 minutes or until almost set. Run a sharp knife around the edge of the cheesecake. Cool in the pan on a wire rack for 30 minutes. Chill, covered, for 4 to 10 hours and cut into wedges.

Yield: 16 servings

NUTRIENTS PER SERVING

Calories	168	Cholesterol	12 mg	Fiber	1 g
Total Fat	6 g	Protein	9 g	Sodium	355 mg
Saturated Fat	2 g	Carbohydrates	20 g	Total Sugar	9 g

DIETARY EXCHANGES: 1 Other Carbohydrate/Sugar, 1 Medium Fat Meat
CARB CHOICES: 1

Heavenly Light Cheesecake

Graham Cracker Crust
3/4 cup graham cracker crumbs
2 tablespoons margarine, melted

Filling
15 ounces part-skim
  ricotta cheese
1 cup plain nonfat yogurt

1 cup Splenda or granulated
  artificial sweetener
2 tablespoons all-purpose flour
2 tablespoons lemon juice
8 ounces light cream
  cheese, softened
3/4 cup liquid egg substitute
2 1/2 teaspoons vanilla extract

For the crust, preheat the oven to 325 degrees. Toss the graham cracker crumbs and margarine in a bowl until coated. Press the crumb mixture over the bottom of a 9-inch springform pan and bake for 5 minutes. Let stand until cool. Maintain the oven temperature.

For the filling, process the ricotta cheese, yogurt, artificial sweetener, flour and lemon juice in a blender until smooth. Beat the cream cheese in a mixing bowl until light and fluffy. Add the egg substitute and vanilla to the cream cheese and beat until blended. Add the ricotta cheese mixture gradually, beating constantly until smooth. Spread the cheese mixture over the baked layer.

Place the pan on a baking sheet and bake for 1 hour or until the center is almost set. Cool on a wire rack for 15 minutes. Run a sharp knife around the edge of the cheesecake to loosen. Cool for 30 minutes longer and remove the side of the pan. Let stand until completely cool. Chill, covered, for 4 to 6 hours before serving.

Yield: 12 servings

NUTRIENTS PER SERVING

Calories	150	Cholesterol	18 mg	Fiber	<1 g
Total Fat	7 g	Protein	9 g	Sodium	207 mg
Saturated Fat	3 g	Carbohydrates	11 g	Total Sugar	4 g

DIETARY EXCHANGES: 1 Milk, 1 Fat
CARB CHOICES: 1

Angel Surprise

1 (16-ounce) can juice-pack fruit cocktail
1 (9-inch) angel food cake
1 teaspoon grated lemon zest
1 envelope unflavored gelatin
1 cup lemon nonfat yogurt
12 ounces nonfat whipped topping

Drain the fruit cocktail, reserving $1/2$ cup of the juice. Cut a 1-inch slice from the top of the cake, reserving the slice. Remove the center of the cake, leaving a 1-inch shell. Mix the reserved juice and lemon zest in a saucepan and sprinkle with the gelatin. Let stand for 1 minute or until softened.

Bring the gelatin mixture to a boil over medium heat and boil for 3 minutes, stirring constantly. Let stand until cool and stir in the yogurt. Spoon into a bowl and chill until slightly thickened.

Combine the fruit cocktail and one-half of the whipped topping in a bowl and mix well. Fold in the gelatin mixture and spoon into the cake shell. Top with the reserved cake slice. Spread the remaining whipped topping over the side and top of the cake. Chill, covered, for 8 hours or longer.

Yield: 12 servings

NUTRIENTS PER SERVING

Calories	159	Cholesterol	<1 mg	Fiber	1 g
Total Fat	<1 g	Protein	3 g	Sodium	245 mg
Saturated Fat	<1 g	Carbohydrates	34 g	Total Sugar	11 g

DIETARY EXCHANGES: 1 Other Carbohydrate/Sugar, 1 Fruit
CARB CHOICES: 2

Apple Spice Cake

5 Granny Smith apples, peeled
  and cut into $1/2$-inch slices
7 tablespoons unsweetened
  apple juice
1 (21-ounce) can no-sugar-
  added apple pie filling
  or topping
1 teaspoon ground cinnamon

1 teaspoon ground nutmeg
1 teaspoon ground allspice
1 tablespoon sugar
1 (2-layer) package spice
  cake mix
$1/2$ cup chopped pecans
3 tablespoons butter
$1/4$ cup light pancake syrup

Arrange the apples in a microwave-safe dish and drizzle with
2 tablespoons of the apple juice. Microwave, covered with plastic wrap,
on High for 5 minutes and stir. Microwave on High for 5 minutes longer
or until the apples are tender. Stir in the pie filling.

Preheat the oven to 350 degrees. Spread the apple mixture in a
9×13-inch cake pan sprayed with nonstick cooking spray. Sprinkle with
a mixture of the cinnamon, nutmeg, allspice and sugar. Spread the dry
cake mix evenly over the top and sprinkle with the pecans.

Combine the remaining 5 tablespoons apple juice, the butter and syrup
in a microwave-safe measuring cup and microwave until the butter melts.
Stir and drizzle the juice mixture over the prepared layers. Bake for 45 to
55 minutes or until brown. Serve warm with frozen yogurt.

Yield: 15 servings

NUTRIENTS PER SERVING

Calories	242	Cholesterol	15 mg	Fiber	2 g
Total Fat	9 g	Protein	3 g	Sodium	295 mg
Saturated Fat	0 g	Carbohydrates	38 g	Total Sugar	25 g

DIETARY EXCHANGES: 1 Other Carbohydrate/Sugar, 1 Fruit, 2 Fat
CARB CHOICES: 2

Applesauce Cake

1 cup raisins
1 cup mixed dried fruit
2 cups water
2 cups all-purpose flour
1 teaspoon ground cinnamon
$1/2$ teaspoon ground nutmeg
1 teaspoon baking soda

$1/2$ teaspoon salt
4 envelopes artificial sweetener
1 cup unsweetened applesauce
$3/4$ cup canola oil
2 eggs, lightly beaten
1 teaspoon vanilla extract

Preheat the oven to 350 degrees. Combine the raisins, dried fruit and water in a saucepan and cook until all of the water is absorbed, stirring occasionally. Let stand until lukewarm. Mix the flour, cinnamon, nutmeg, baking soda, salt and artificial sweetener in a bowl. Stir in the applesauce, canola oil, eggs and vanilla. Blend in the raisin mixture.

Spoon the batter into a greased 10-inch tube pan or bundt pan and bake for 35 to 40 minutes or until the cake tests done. Cool in the pan for 10 minutes and invert onto a wire rack to cool completely.

Yield: 16 servings

NUTRIENTS PER SERVING

Calories	222	Cholesterol	26 mg	Fiber	2 g
Total Fat	11 g	Protein	3 g	Sodium	162 mg
Saturated Fat	1 g	Carbohydrates	28 g	Total Sugar	12 g

DIETARY EXCHANGES: 1 Starch, 1 Fruit, 2 Fat
CARB CHOICES: 2

IF YOU WANT THE RAINBOW, YOU GOTTA
PUT UP WITH THE RAIN.

—STEVEN WRIGHT

Strawberry Yogurt Cake

1 (2-layer) package white cake mix
$3/4$ cup water
2 egg whites
$1/3$ cup unsweetened applesauce
2 cups strawberry low-fat or fat-free yogurt
8 ounces lite whipped topping
Fresh strawberries, cut into halves for garnish

Preheat the oven to 350 degrees. Combine the cake mix, water, egg whites and applesauce in a bowl and mix until blended. Stir in 1 cup of the yogurt. Spread the batter in a 9×13-inch cake pan sprayed with nonstick cooking spray. Bake for 30 minutes or until the cake tests done. Cool in the pan on a wire rack.

Mix the remaining 1 cup yogurt and the whipped topping in a bowl and spread over the top of the cake. Chill, covered, until serving time. Slice the cake and garnish each serving with fresh strawberries.

Yield: 15 servings

NUTRIENTS PER SERVING

Calories	221	Cholesterol	1 mg	Fiber	<1 g
Total Fat	6 g	Protein	4 g	Sodium	259 mg
Saturated Fat	2 g	Carbohydrates	39 g	Total Sugar	28 g

DIETARY EXCHANGES: 1 Starch, 1 Other Carbohydrate/Sugar, 1 Fat
CARB CHOICES: 2

Banana Apple Bread

2 cups all-purpose flour
2 teaspoons baking powder
1 teaspoon baking soda
$1/2$ teaspoon salt
2 very ripe bananas, mashed
2 eggs
$1/4$ cup honey

1 teaspoon vanilla extract
1 teaspoon ground allspice
1 teaspoon ground cinnamon
$1/3$ cup raisins
2 Granny Smith apples, peeled
   and chopped

Preheat the oven to 375 degrees. Mix the flour, baking powder, baking soda and salt together. Combine the bananas, eggs, honey, vanilla, allspice and cinnamon in a mixing bowl and beat until blended. Add the flour mixture and mix just until moistened. Fold in the raisins and apples.

Spoon the batter into a greased and floured 5×9-inch loaf pan and bake for 40 to 45 minutes or until the loaf tests done. Cool in the pan for 10 minutes and invert onto a wire rack to cool completely.

Yield: 12 slices

NUTRIENTS PER SLICE

Calories	150	Cholesterol	35 mg	Fiber	2 g
Total Fat	1 g	Protein	4 g	Sodium	296 mg
Saturated Fat	<1 g	Carbohydrates	32 g	Total Sugar	13 g

DIETARY EXCHANGES: 1 Starch, 1 Fruit
CARB CHOICES: 2

BEFORE EVERYTHING ELSE, GETTING READY
IS THE SECRET OF SUCCESS.

—HENRY FORD

Pineapple Muffins

Muffins
$2^{1/2}$ cups all-purpose flour
2 teaspoons baking powder
1 teaspoon baking soda
$1/2$ teaspoon salt
$1/2$ cup (1 stick) butter, softened
3 eggs
1 cup unsweetened
   pineapple juice
1 teaspoon lemon juice

1 cup drained crushed pineapple
$1/2$ cup ground pecans

Pineapple Frosting
8 ounces fat-free cream
   cheese, softened
2 tablespoons butter, softened
2 tablespoons drained
   crushed pineapple

For the muffins, preheat the oven to 350 degrees. Mix the flour, baking powder, baking soda and salt together. Combine the butter and eggs in a mixing bowl and beat until light and fluffy. Add the pineapple juice and lemon juice and mix until blended. Beat in the flour mixture until smooth and stir in the pineapple and pecans.

Fill fourteen paper-lined muffin cups two-thirds full. Bake at 350 degrees for 20 minutes or until the muffins test done. Remove to a wire rack to cool.

For the frosting, beat the cream cheese and butter in a mixing bowl until light and fluffy. Stir in the pineapple. Spread the frosting over the tops of the cooled muffins.

Yield: 14 muffins

NUTRIENTS PER MUFFIN

Calories	228	Cholesterol	68 mg	Fiber	1 g
Total Fat	12 g	Protein	7 g	Sodium	405 mg
Saturated Fat	6 g	Carbohydrates	24 g	Total Sugar	5 g

DIETARY EXCHANGES: 1 Starch, 1 Fruit, 2 Fat
CARB CHOICES: 2

Brownie Oat Cookies

1 cup quick-cooking oats
$2/3$ cup all-purpose flour
$1/3$ cup sugar
$1/3$ cup Splenda
$1/4$ cup baking cocoa
1 teaspoon baking powder
2 egg whites, lightly beaten
$1/3$ cup light corn syrup
1 teaspoon vanilla extract

Preheat the oven to 350 degrees. Combine the oats, flour, sugar, artificial sweetener, baking cocoa and baking powder in a bowl and mix well. Add the egg whites, corn syrup and vanilla and mix just until moistened.

Drop by teaspoonfuls onto a cookie sheet sprayed with nonstick cooking spray and bake for 10 minutes or until set. Cool on the cookie sheet for 2 minutes and remove to a wire rack to cool completely. Store in an airtight container.

Yield: 24 cookies

NUTRIENTS PER COOKIE

Calories	55	Cholesterol	0 mg	Fiber	1 g
Total Fat	<1 g	Protein	1 g	Sodium	28 mg
Saturated Fat	<1 g	Carbohydrates	12 g	Total Sugar	4 g

DIETARY EXCHANGES: 1 Other Carbohydrate/Sugar
CARB CHOICES: 1

IT'S EASIER TO GO DOWN A HILL THAN UP IT, BUT
THE VIEW IS MUCH BETTER AT THE TOP.

—HENRY WARD BEECHER

Honey and Banana Scones

PHOTOGRAPH FOR THIS RECIPE APPEARS ON PAGE 86.

1 cup all-purpose flour
1 tablespoon baking powder
1 teaspoon salt
1 cup whole wheat flour
2 tablespoons butter

$1/2$ cup skim milk
2 tablespoons honey
2 bananas, mashed
1 tablespoon skim milk

Preheat the oven to 450 degrees. Sift the all-purpose flour, baking powder and salt into a bowl and mix well. Stir in the whole wheat flour and cut in the butter until crumbly. Make a well in the center of the flour mixture. Mix $1/2$ cup skim milk and the honey in a bowl and add to the well, stirring until blended. Mix in the bananas with a fork.

Knead the dough several times on a lightly floured surface. Divide the dough into two equal portions. Roll or pat each portion into a $3/4$-inch-thick round and cut each round into eight wedges.

Arrange the wedges $1 1/2$ inches apart on a baking sheet sprayed with nonstick cooking spray. Brush the tops with 1 tablespoon skim milk and bake for 10 to 12 minutes or until light brown. Cool on the baking sheet for 2 minutes and remove to a wire rack. Cool for 3 minutes longer and serve warm. You may cut the dough into rounds instead of wedges, if desired.

Yield: 16 scones

NUTRIENTS PER SCONE

Calories	91	Cholesterol	4 mg	Fiber	2 g
Total Fat	2 g	Protein	2 g	Sodium	251 mg
Saturated Fat	1 g	Carbohydrates	18 g	Total Sugar	5 g

DIETARY EXCHANGES: 1 Starch
CARB CHOICES: 1

Miniature Cream Puffs

1 cup water
1/2 cup (1 stick) butter
1/4 teaspoon salt
1 cup all-purpose flour

4 eggs
1 large package sugar-free
fat-free chocolate instant
pudding mix, prepared

Preheat the oven to 400 degrees. Bring the water, butter and salt to a rolling boil in a saucepan over high heat, stirring occasionally. Reduce the heat to low and stir in the flour. Cook until the mixture leaves the side of the pan, stirring constantly with a wooden spoon. Remove from the heat.

Add the eggs one at a time, mixing until smooth and glossy after each addition. Drop by spoonfuls onto an ungreased baking sheet and bake for 10 minutes. Reduce the oven temperature to 350 degrees and bake for 15 minutes longer or until golden brown and firm. Split the cream puffs and remove the soft dough. Fill with equal amounts of the pudding.

Yield: 36 cream puffs

NUTRIENTS PER CREAM PUFF

Calories	56	Cholesterol	30 mg	Fiber	<1 g
Total Fat	3 g	Protein	2 g	Sodium	107 mg
Saturated Fat	2 g	Carbohydrates	5 g	Total Sugar	1 g

DIETARY EXCHANGES: 1 Fat
CARB CHOICES: 0

TIME MAY BE A GREAT HEALER, BUT IT'S
ALSO A LOUSY BEAUTICIAN.

Chocolate Cream Cheese Pie

$1/2$ cup Grape-Nuts cereal
4 teaspoons reduced-calorie margarine
8 ounces fat-free cream cheese, softened
1 cup fat-free sour cream
1 small package sugar-free chocolate
  instant pudding mix
8 tablespoons whipped cream

Preheat the oven to 350 degrees. Mix the cereal and margarine in a bowl and pat into a 9-inch pie plate. Bake for 10 minutes. Let stand until cool.

Beat the cream cheese, sour cream and pudding mix in a mixing bowl until blended. Spread the cream cheese mixture over the baked layer and chill or freeze until set. Slice the pie and top each serving with 1 tablespoon of the whipped topping.

Yield: 8 servings

NUTRIENTS PER SERVING

Calories	116	Cholesterol	10 mg	Fiber	1 g
Total Fat	3 g	Protein	7 g	Sodium	306 mg
Saturated Fat	1 g	Carbohydrates	16 g	Total Sugar	6 g

DIETARY EXCHANGES: 1 Milk
CARB CHOICES: 1

No-Bake Creamy Pumpkin Pie

1 cup skim milk
2 small packages sugar-free vanilla
  instant pudding mix
$1^1/2$ teaspoons pumpkin pie spice
1 (15-ounce) can pumpkin purée
1 (9-inch) graham cracker pie shell
1 cup nonfat whipped topping

Combine the skim milk, pudding mix and pumpkin pie spice in a bowl and mix until blended. Stir in the pumpkin until smooth.

Spread the pumpkin filling in the pie shell and spread with the whipped topping. Chill, covered, in the refrigerator for up to 2 days.

Yield: 8 servings

NUTRIENTS PER SERVING

Calories	155	Cholesterol	1 mg	Fiber	3 g
Total Fat	5 g	Protein	3 g	Sodium	424 mg
Saturated Fat	1 g	Carbohydrates	26 g	Total Sugar	9 g

DIETARY EXCHANGES: 1 Starch, 1 Other Carbohydrate/Sugar
CARB CHOICES: 2

> I DON'T CARE WHAT IS WRITTEN ABOUT ME
> AS LONG AS IT ISN'T TRUE.
>
> —KATHARINE HEPBURN

Strawberry Pie

1 small package sugar-free vanilla
  instant pudding mix
1 small package sugar-free strawberry gelatin
$2^1/2$ cups cold water
4 cups sliced strawberries
1 (9-inch) graham cracker pie shell
Nonfat whipped topping for garnish

Mix the pudding mix, gelatin and cold water in a saucepan and bring to a boil over medium heat, stirring constantly. Remove from the heat and cool slightly. Chill until slightly thickened.

Arrange the strawberries in the pie shell. Pour the gelatin mixture over the top. Chill until set. Garnish each slice with a dollop of whipped topping.

Yield: 8 servings

NUTRIENTS PER SERVING

Calories	150	Cholesterol	0 mg	Fiber	2 g
Total Fat	6 g	Protein	1 g	Sodium	242 mg
Saturated Fat	1 g	Carbohydrates	23 g	Total Sugar	10 g

DIETARY EXCHANGES: 1 Other Carbohydrate/Sugar, 1 Fat
CARB CHOICES: 1

Baking Equivalents

	When the recipe calls for	Use
Baking	$1/2$ cup (1 stick) butter 2 cups (4 sticks) butter 4 cups all-purpose flour $41/2$ cups sifted cake flour 1 square chocolate 1 cup semisweet chocolate chips 4 cups marshmallows $21/4$ cups packed brown sugar 4 cups confectioners' sugar 2 cups sugar	4 ounces 1 pound 1 pound 1 pound 1 ounce 6 ounces 1 pound 1 pound 1 pound 1 pound
Cereal/Bread	1 cup fine dry bread crumbs 1 cup soft bread crumbs 1 cup small bread crumbs 1 cup fine saltine crumbs 1 cup fine graham cracker crumbs 1 cup vanilla wafer crumbs 1 cup crushed cornflakes 4 cups cooked macaroni $31/2$ cups cooked rice	4 to 5 slices 2 slices 2 slices 28 saltines 15 graham crackers 22 wafers 3 cups uncrushed 8 ounces uncooked 1 cup uncooked
Dairy	1 cup shredded cheese 1 cup cottage cheese 1 cup sour cream 1 cup whipped cream $2/3$ cup evaporated milk $12/3$ cups evaporated milk	4 ounces 8 ounces 8 ounces $1/2$ cup heavy cream 1 ($51/3$-ounce) can 1 (13-ounce) can

Fruit	4 cups sliced or chopped apples
	1 cup mashed bananas
	2 cups pitted cherries
	$21/2$ cups shredded coconut
	4 cups cranberries
	1 cup pitted dates
	1 cup candied fruit
	3 to 4 tablespoons lemon juice plus
	    1 tablespoon grated lemon zest
	$1/3$ cup orange juice plus 2 teaspoons
	    grated orange zest
	4 cups sliced peaches
	2 cups pitted prunes
	3 cups raisins
		4 medium
		3 medium
		4 cups unpitted
		8 ounces
		1 pound
		1 (8-ounce) package
		1 (8-ounce) package
		1 lemon
		
		1 orange
		
		8 medium
		1 (12-ounce) package
		1 (15-ounce) package

Basic Substitutions

	If the recipe calls for	You can substitute
Flour	1 cup sifted all-purpose flour	1 cup less 2 tablespoons unsifted all-purpose flour
	1 cup sifted cake flour	1 cup less 2 tablespoons sifted all-purpose flour
	1 cup sifted self-rising flour	1 cup sifted all-purpose flour plus $1\frac{1}{2}$ teaspoons baking powder and a pinch of salt
Milk/Cream	1 cup buttermilk	1 cup plain yogurt, or 1 tablespoon lemon juice or vinegar plus enough milk to measure 1 cup—let stand for 5 minutes before using
	1 cup whipping cream or half-and-half	$\frac{7}{8}$ cup whole milk plus $1\frac{1}{2}$ tablespoons butter
	1 cup light cream	$\frac{7}{8}$ cup whole milk plus 3 tablespoons butter
	1 cup sour milk	1 cup plain yogurt
	1 cup whole milk	1 cup skim or nonfat milk plus 2 tablespoons butter or margarine
Seasonings	1 teaspoon allspice	$\frac{1}{2}$ teaspoon cinnamon plus $\frac{1}{8}$ teaspoon cloves
	1 teaspoon Italian spice	$\frac{1}{4}$ teaspoon each oregano, basil, thyme, rosemary plus dash of cayenne pepper
	1 teaspoon lemon juice	$\frac{1}{2}$ teaspoon vinegar
Sugar	1 cup confectioners' sugar	$\frac{1}{2}$ cup plus 1 tablespoon granulated sugar
	1 cup granulated sugar	$1\frac{3}{4}$ cups confectioners' sugar, 1 cup packed light brown sugar or $\frac{3}{4}$ cup honey
Other	1 package active dry yeast	$\frac{1}{2}$ cake compressed yeast
	1 teaspoon baking powder	$\frac{1}{4}$ teaspoon cream of tartar plus $\frac{1}{4}$ teaspoon baking soda
	1 cup dry bread crumbs	$\frac{3}{4}$ cup cracker crumbs or 1 cup cornflake crumbs
	1 cup (2 sticks) butter	$\frac{7}{8}$ cup vegetable oil or 1 cup margarine
	1 tablespoon cornstarch	2 tablespoons all-purpose flour
	$1\frac{2}{3}$ ounces semisweet chocolate	1 ounce unsweetened chocolate plus 4 teaspoons granulated sugar
	1 ounce unsweetened chocolate	3 tablespoons unsweetened baking cocoa plus 1 tablespoon butter or margarine
	1 cup honey	1 to $1\frac{1}{4}$ cups sugar plus $\frac{1}{4}$ cup liquid, or 1 cup corn syrup or molasses
	1 egg	$\frac{1}{4}$ cup mayonnaise

Refrigeration Guidelines

Food	Refrigerate	Freeze
Beef steaks	1 to 2 days	6 to 12 months
Beef roasts	1 to 2 days	6 to 12 months
Corned beef	7 days	2 weeks
Pork chops	1 to 2 days	3 to 4 months
Pork roasts	1 to 2 days	4 to 8 months
Fresh sausage	1 to 2 days	1 to 2 months
Smoked sausage	7 days	Not recommended
Cured ham	5 to 7 days	1 to 2 months
Canned ham	1 year	Not recommended
Sliced ham	3 days	1 to 2 months
Bacon	7 days	2 to 4 months
Veal cutlets	1 to 2 days	6 to 9 months
Stew meat	1 to 2 days	3 to 4 months
Ground meat	1 to 2 days	3 to 4 months
Luncheon meats	3 to 5 days	Not recommended
Frankfurters	7 days	1 month
Whole chicken	1 to 2 days	12 months
Chicken pieces	1 to 2 days	9 months

Freezing Tips

- List the date on all items before placing them in the freezer.

- Freezing canned hams or processed meats is not recommended. Frozen canned hams become watery and soft when thawed. Processed meats have a high salt content, which speeds rancidity when thawed.

- Do not freeze stuffed chickens or turkeys. The stuffing may incur bacterial contamination during the lengthy thawing process.

- Partially thawed food that still has ice crystals in the package can be safely refrozen. A safer test is to determine if the surface temperature is 40 degrees Fahrenheit or lower.

Index

Index

Index

Index